THE PROSTATE

The Prostate

Everything You Need to Know
about the Man Gland

Yosh Taguchi, M.D.
Introduction by Adrian Waller, Ph.D.

KEY PORTER ✎ **BOOKS**

Canadian Cataloguing in Publication Data

Taguchi, Yosh, 1933–
    The Prostate: everything you need to know about the man gland

Includes index.
ISBN 1-55263-277-6

1. Prostate—Diseases—Popular works. I. Title.

RC899.T33 2000   616.6'5   C00-931702-3

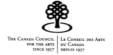

The Canada Council   Le Conseil des Arts
For the Arts   du Canada
Since 1957   Depuis 1957

The publisher gratefully acknowledges the support of the Canada Council for the Arts and the Ontario Arts Council for its publishing program.

We acknowledge the financial support of the Government of Canada through the Book Publishing Industry Development Program (BPIDP) for our publishing activities.

Key Porter Books Limited
70 The Esplanade
Toronto, Ontario
Canada M5E 1R2

www.keyporter.com

Design: Peter Maher
Electronic formatting: Heidy Lawrance Associates

Publisher's Note: The contents of this book are not intended to be used as a substitution for consultation with your physician. All matters pertaining to your health should be directed to a health care professional.

Printed and bound in Canada

01 02 03 04 05 6 5 4 3 2 1

*For my wife, Joan, who gave me invaluable
support while I was long preoccupied with my
profession, and who raised with me four children,
our source of pride and joy:
Kathleen, Edwin, Jocelyn, and Carolin.
Also for my late friend Marcel Einhorn,
who introduced me to tennis
and improved my health.
May he rest in peace.*

Contents

Introduction

I first heard about Yosh Taguchi in a swimming pool near Fort Lauderdale, Florida, in February 1999. No name ever sounded sweeter.

By then I'd suffered through a history of urinary tract problems that included numerous bladder infections, two operations to alleviate prostate enlargement, and a lot of discomfort and anxiety in between. I had had my latest operation only a month or so before standing in that pool: I had been diagnosed with prostate cancer. The problem was, who should I turn to for help?

I read many books on the subject and acquainted myself with my options. In light of my medical history, however, I needed an understanding urologist who could prescribe what was best for me, and quickly. At sixty-two, after all, I was still relatively young; I yearned to be tumor-free without all the side effects that prostate cancer patients are known to endure.

One of the swimmers in the pool that warm afternoon was a fifty-one-year-old Montreal developer who had also suffered his fair share of prostate ailments.

"If you live in Canada," he said, "you shouldn't look any further than a guy named Yosh Taguchi. Give him a call. Tell him I sent you. I'm a friend of his."

"A friend? Really?"

"Well, he sorted me out magnificently when I couldn't piss properly for months on end, and I know several guys he's cured of cancer. You'll like him."

Two or three days later, and by sheer coincidence, my wife mentioned my dilemma to yet another Montrealer who, like me, had made Florida his second home. He uttered two words.

"Yosh Taguchi."

"That's what someone else has suggested," I said.

"Don't fiddle about," the man said, "and don't worry. If you live most of the time in Montreal you should give Yosh a call. He's wonderful. He'll fix you up in no time. Old Yosh fixes everyone up. That's why he's on radio all the time, talking about it. He's a very special man. Tell him I referred you. I'm a friend of his."

"You're a friend, too?"

"Yep."

That day, I called Yosh Taguchi's secretary and made an appointment to see him. He examined me for the first time on my return to Montreal that March, and the rest is history. He advised me to have my prostate removed and I agreed. Dr. Taguchi performed the operation at Montreal's Royal Victoria Hospital six weeks later, and I have been cancer-free ever since.

A minor side effect, however—tissue scarring where the urethra meets the bladder—resulted, and as I lay on an operating table, waiting for Yosh Taguchi to appear to treat this, I could not help but joke with the most senior urology nurse.

"Is this guy *really* the best there is for this procedure?" I asked. "I mean, if he isn't tell me now and I'll get dressed and go home!"

"Are you kidding?" the nurse responded. "Dr. Taguchi is the best urologist in Canada."

At that, there was a general chorus of approval, and a voice came at me from an adjacent room. It belonged to a resident who was scrubbing up to assist in my treatment.

"You're all wrong, wrong, wrong!" the resident said. "Dr. Yosh Taguchi is one of the best urologists in the world!"

Not being a physician, I cannot substantiate this opinion from any medical viewpoint. In any case, there are numerous capable urologists in Canada who do excellent work, and some of these earn international stature, too. What I *can* say, however, is that during that apprehensive wait for the first major operation I had ever had—a radical prostatectomy—I shared my thoughts with my wife's friend Dr. Jacques Abourbih, a respected urologist in Sudbury, Ontario.

"Who's actually doing your surgery?" Dr. Abourbih asked.

"Yosh Taguchi," I said.

"You are very lucky," Dr. Abourbih added. "Yosh Taguchi was my mentor. He taught me so much of what I practice today. His knowledge about the prostate and his skill in fixing it when it goes wrong are absolutely unsurpassed. You are in excellent hands."

I thought I was, especially when Jacques Abourbih revealed a side of the affable, smiling Yosh Taguchi that few of his patients ever get to know—the meticulousness of his medical reading and diagnostics, and his work in the operating theater. In a career spanning some four decades, he has performed more than 500 radical prostatectomies and still confides that he wants to make each better than the previous one—that his entire being is consumed with honing his surgical skills so as to achieve what he calls "the absolute-perfect surgical procedure."

It's no secret that Yosh Taguchi and I have become friends. We really have. Once, when we were dining in a restaurant near Miami—after having spent a day together discussing our respective professions—Yosh asked me where I had first heard about him. I jumped at the chance to recall the man in the swimming pool and the other former patient I had met later.

Yosh smiled as he remembered how each new patient is invariably referred to him not by a family practitioner, but by "a friend."

"I never knew how many friends I had until I started treating prostates," he quipped, "but I have to tell you that the journey has been truly wonderful."

I think it has, and this comforting book, with its advice, detail, and wisdom, will attest to it.

Adrian Waller, Ph.D.
Montreal, 2000

Author's note

In this book I discuss the three main prostate ailments:

- prostate enlargement
- prostatitis (inflammation of the prostate gland)
- cancer

These are the diseases that reinforce the notion that, for its weight and size, the prostate is the source of more health problems than any other part of the male anatomy.

Along the way, I describe what we have come to know about prostate function, what is still not clear to us, and what is purely conjectural. I also describe what treatments are available and how I have applied them.

Whenever I mention drugs I use their better-known trade names. Where necessary, I give the usual dosages so that they can be brought up for discussion, and I offer some practical advice on what drugs are best for what prostate ailments.

Long a taboo subject, the prostate gland has at last become "mentionable" and has engendered numerous publications. Thus, when Anna Porter (publisher of Key Porter Books) asked me if I would write about it for the general public, I wondered if I could add anything worthwhile to what had already been written. I figured a popular book on the prostate would have to appeal first to those patients who have been newly diagnosed with prostate disorders, and then to the men who are likely to be affected by these problems as time goes on. Of course, the book would have to appeal to the readers' partners, as well.

The questions were: Could I write a book that would appeal to all three populations? Should I aim for one population at the expense of the others?

I pondered a medical dilemma, too. If I strove for too much simplicity in discussing a subject that is, in fact, highly complex, I might upset my colleagues. Could I possibly write a book that was both comprehensive and comprehensible?

With the help of my friend, the Canadian writer Adrian Waller, I decided to write a book that would be understood by as many people as possible. My aim was to try to reproduce a text that would work as well as my previous effort, *Private Parts* (McClelland & Stewart), which was enormously successful in Canada and was subsequently translated into five other languages—French, Spanish, Japanese, Chinese, and Russian. This book also went into second editions in English and French. The appeal, I think, was in its simplicity, clarity, and honesty.

There are, of course, many books on prostate diseases. For prostate cancer specifically, there are a number of textbooks meant for students, doctors, and other professionals, but the technical jargon of most of these generally turns most patients off.

Recently, the *Canadian Medical Association Journal* ran a series of papers on prostate cancer and then compiled the articles into a book entitled *Prostate Cancer: Balancing the Risks in Diagnosis and Treatment*. It is meant for doctors, but the style is such that many patients may also find it useful.

Then, there are books for the public written by recognized authorities: Patrick Walsh's *The Prostate: A Guide for Men and the Women Who Love Them*, for instance, which contains a lot of useful information.

A number of prostate cancer patients have also written books about their ordeals. Cornelius Ryan, famous for such novels as *A Bridge Too Far* and *The Longest Day*, may have been the first. In *A Private Battle*, he directs quite a lot of anger toward certain surgeons and institutions. Michael Korda, editor in chief at Simon & Schuster (and the editor of Ryan's book), chronicled his own battle in *Man to Man: Surviving Prostate Cancer*.

I found Korda's account gripping and honest, although, he, too, faults urologists for their arrogance and seeming indifference to his suffering.

James Lewis has become something of a patient advocate with his book *How I Survived Prostate Cancer ... And So Can You*. He pulls no punches, and I applaud him for the effort. A subsequent edition, *New Guidelines for Surviving Prostate Cancer*, was released in 1997 and is very much up-to-date.

Audrey Newton, another Canadian, wrote a book about her husband's battle, entitled *Living with Prostate Cancer*. It is a moving account and I was pleased to be asked to write a foreword to it.

One of my own patients, René Delbuguet, wrote a book in French called *Ma prostate chérie*. I read the English translation, and found it captivating and entertaining. Certainly, it brings home to practicing physicians the burden we place on the patient population when we ask them to participate in their choice of treatments.

Today, it would appear that doctors can abandon responsibility for making hard decisions. They can hide behind practice guidelines and *ad hoc* decisions. Doctors are a privileged lot. They may have had to study hard and long, but it is society that has borne the bulk of the costs for producing these highly skilled men and women.

Medical school fees represent just 10 percent of the cost of producing a medical doctor. A specialist has spent four years in high school, four years in undergraduate university studies, four years in medical school, and five years in specialty training. Does it make sense for patients to make critical decisions for themselves after a five-minute lecture and an evening's exposure to the Internet?

In my view, doctors need to make the tough calls—whether it is to carry out an operation or to turn off a respirator. That is what they have been trained to do.

So much for philosophy. It goes without saying that in this book I have tried to explain prostate gland problems as simply as possible. It is my hope that this approach will make what I have to say relevant to a lot of people—men and their partners alike.

Yosh Taguchi, M.D.
Montreal, 2000

1. The nature of the beast

Not long ago, one of the hundred or so patients I see each week at Montreal's Royal Victoria Hospital asked me, "Why do I have a prostate, doc?"

Although I have been practicing urology for almost forty years, I was a little taken aback by his question. No one had ever asked it of me before.

"I mean," the patient went on, "I know why I've got an elbow, a thyroid, and a penis, and I know they're all useful. But no doctor has yet been able to tell me why I have a prostate. Oh, they can all tell me the problems I'm having with my prostate, but I'm still waiting for one of them to explain why I have this gland in the first place. What does it do? What is it there for? Can I live without it?"

I thought for a moment before telling the patient exactly what I have been telling my students at McGill University, where I have been lecturing for as long as I've been practicing: This small, walnut-sized gland that sits at the neck of the blad-der where it meets the urethra, behind the pubic bone, and in front of the rectum, weighing a mere 20 grams when it is healthy, has a very limited use—which, as we will find out, diminishes as a man ages.

It is needed most when a man is in his younger years and wants to impregnate a woman, or when he is merely seeking to exercise his sexual prowess. Nonetheless, the prostate gland is not a "prostitute" gland, as another of my patients used to refer to it. Nor is it the "prostrate," which is how less-aware men and women referred to it before the gland found itself at the center of so many news reports.

To remember the difference, I used to tell my medical students, "The man lay prostrate in his bed waiting for the doctor to examine his prostate." They quickly saw the difference and laughed. Prostate problems, however, are no laughing matter at all—and those students knew it all too well.

Normal Male Anatomy

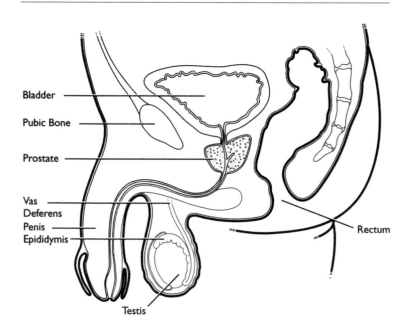

In a young boy, the gland is vestigial or undetectable—almost nonexistent—lying like a cluster of seeds under the lining of the urinary tract. Most boys, I venture to say, don't even know they have the beginnings of a prostate gland that may grow to haunt them later.

At puberty, though, this anatomy begins to change. The surge of the male hormone testosterone stimulates these seeds to germinate and grow. The boy's external sex organs—the penis, the testicles, and the scrotum—also enlarge under the influence of the male hormone at this time, as he finally becomes a man. Now he has a prostate gland.

In essence, the development of this gland resembles the growth of a softwood tree with many branches. Because of this similarity, the growing process has been called "arborization," a term borrowed from botanists. Twenty such "trees" may be involved in this process, but a closer look at the end result suggests that the growth more closely resembles a patch of raspberry bushes.

Little glandular structures (called *acini* by the pathologists) within the larger prostate represent the berries, while the muscular supporting tissue, called *stroma*, make up the stem and leaves. In a normal prostate, the glandular component comprises 20 percent, and the muscle cells 40 percent, of the total mass.

Remember this raspberry bush analogy—I will come back to it later when I discuss prostate enlargement and, of course, the much more serious ailment, prostate cancer, the dread of every man alive.

Thankfully, most men never get this awful disease, but statistical evidence does not prevent them from thinking unceasingly about what may happen to their prostate glands as they age. In fact, it is true to say that almost all males over forty worry now and then about this part of their anatomy, and

Formation of the Prostate

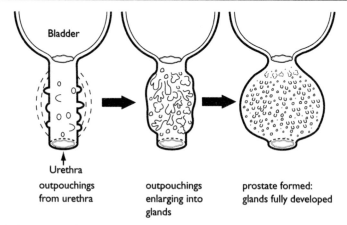

| outpouchings from urethra | outpouchings enlarging into glands | prostate formed: glands fully developed |

while a lot of this worry is disease-related, a good part of it may be purely psychological.

The prostate gland produces a protein called prostate specific antigen (PSA), about which you will hear a lot. When spermatozoa from the testicles and a jelly-like substance from the seminal vesicles flow into the prostate, they join up with the PSA and other prostatic secretions to make what we know as the ejaculate fluid. Later, the PSA transforms that sticky substance into a distinctly liquid form, which is important in the fertilization process.

Actually, the prostate secretes 60 percent of the ejaculate. Or, to put it another way, it makes the bulk of the fluid in which the spermatozoa—or the sperm ejaculated on orgasm— are contained.

This prostatic fluid, however, is not essential for sperm maturation or sperm survival. In fact, sperm extracted from the epididymis, where it exits from the testicle, can create a normal pregnancy on its own without needing to pass through the prostate. So, neither the PSA nor the seminal vesicles found on either side of the gland actually need to figure in the fertilization process. We know, for example, that we can draw sperm directly from the testicle or epididymis by syringe for impregnation, long before it even reaches the prostate. This, in fact, is what is done in assisted reproduction.

Nonetheless, it is vital for the sperm to be in this medium when natural impregnation is the goal. Ironically, then, when a man reaches middle age and no longer wants to impregnate a woman, he really has no further use for this gland, yet it can cause him more mental anguish, more emotional aggravation—indeed, more bitterness and anger—than any other part of his body.

Accordingly, millions of men the world over ask their urologists the same questions:

- Will my prostate grow and choke my urine flow?
- Will it become cancerous?
- Will surgery or radiotherapy become necessary and leave me wetting the bed or unable to get an erection, or both?
- Will the diagnosis of cancer be missed and lead me to live my life in excruciating pain?
- Will the cancer spread into my bones?
- Will the doctors bungle the job of curing me, no matter what the problem?
- Will my prostate eventually kill me, like my uncle's killed him?
- How can I protect myself from the most severe protate problems?

The root cause of many of the problems that afflict the gland can be found in its design, which is flawed indeed. Ideally, the prostate should have been given an external drainage pipe—such as one fitted to a testicle or a salivary gland—that would help any unwanted inflammation or infection drain away naturally. Unfortunately, this doesn't exist.

If it were a globular gland with an external drainage system, its enlargement would not choke the urinary passage

Prostate Gland Structure

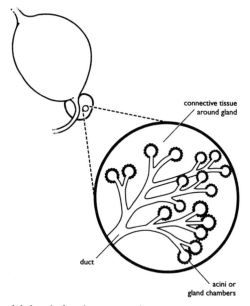

connective tissue
around gland

duct

acini or
gland chambers

and could be left alone, and any cancerous growth could simply be snipped out easily without the need for major reconstructive surgery. Instead, the prostate gland is wrapped *around* the urethra, with an *internal* drainage pipe that is joined by the sperm duct close to its opening, and this means that rather delicate surgery may be required to repair a severely diseased prostate.

As some men who have had their prostate gland removed can testify, it is truly an organ one can live without. This means that, providing there are no other urinary problems involved, a man who doesn't have a prostate can still enjoy life to its fullest, with relatively few side effects. This may come as a surprise to many people, but, like a lot of the men on whom I have performed this radical operation, I can vouch that it is true.

I routinely ask all of my patients who have had their cancerous prostates removed, "Surely there must be some subtle way your life is different now compared to what it was before the surgery?"

Usually, they look at me puzzled and reply, "No, doc. There's really no difference."

Indeed, without a prostate gland, urination can be just as normal, a sex life just as satisfactory, an orgasm just as intense. Much less fluid, however, is ejaculated—which is what I meant when I said that most middle-aged men did not really need the prostate to function as nature had originally intended it. In this way, the prostate can be a tenacious little beast, and, when enlarged or inflamed, the source of a disproportionate amount of distress.

Finally, please remember PSA. The increased production of this protein is used as a marker both for the diagnosis of cancer and for the possible reoccurrence of it after treatment. You will find that as this book progresses, I will refer to it often.

2. Examining the prostate

The term "prostate" comes from the Greek *prostates,* which means "one that stands before." Did the Greeks think that the prostate "stood" before the bladder? Or did they mean that it preceded the penis? Whatever was intended, it seems that the Greeks were almost as uncertain about this enigmatic and inaccessible gland then as we are today.

If you go to a doctor with a sore finger, toe, or elbow, he can see it, touch it, even squeeze it if necessary. He can examine it in such a fashion as to be fairly certain what is wrong with it and what should be done to treat it. The prostate, however, is a different matter. Because it is so deeply set within the pelvic area, it often requires more than one diagnostic procedure to ascertain what ails it.

Consider the three blind men who were asked to describe an elephant. The first felt the tusks and described the animal as being rock hard. The second stroked the elephant's legs and thought the animal was tough and rough. The third felt its ears and thought the animal was soft and velvety. The story tells us that if we rely on only one method of examination, we can make similar errors in judgment.

There are a number of ways we urologists examine the prostate:

- the digital rectal examination
- the cystoscopy
- various imaging techniques, such as the transrectal ultrasound examination, the computerized tomogram scan (CT scan), and the nuclear magnetic scan
- a blood test that identifies the PSA levels

We are also guided by what the patient tells us about his family history, his occupation, and his medical problems—and what he may say in any one of several standardized questionnaires that are used to elicit more specific diagnostic information. These forms invariably ask about the quality and regularity of the patient's urination, if his urine is discolored or foul-smelling (which may denote an infection), how many times he urinates in the night, how easy it is for him to start the flow or stop it, and if he is able to have an erection.

We may also use techniques to measure a patient's actual urine flow and bladder function—tests called "urodynamic studies." These, however, usually come after the more standard investigative procedures have been completed.

When cancer is detected, even more examining techniques are used, and I will discuss these in their appropriate places. For now, I will concentrate on the basic tests that either should be done as a matter of routine, or are administered for diagnosis when a patient complains that he is not urinating properly or is feeling prostatic pain.

The digital rectal examination

For this exam, the doctor places his or her gloved and lubricated index finger into the rectum and feels the back surface of the prostate through the rectum's front wall.

The Canadian Medical Association guidelines for family doctors do not consider this test mandatory. General Norman Schwartzkopf, commander of Desert Storm, must be forever grateful that his physician, an American, was not subject to the same guidelines—it was the digital rectal examination that detected his early prostate cancer. Today, the general is walking testimony to the fact that blood tests alone are often not enough to detect prostate problems; the earliest signs are often detected with the rectal examination, which all men over the age of fifty should have at least once a year.

When performing the test, doctors will either have the patient lie on his side, curled up in the fetal position, or ask him to assume a position wherein his elbows, chest, and knees are on the examining table. I, and many other urologists, prefer to do the rectal exam with the patient standing, feet apart, bent forward, with his elbows on the table. It is, perhaps, a crude position, but I find that it provides the fullest possible access to the gland.

Once the patient is in position, I place my lubricated index finger flat against the anus, which causes the sphincter to relax. When I feel this relaxation, I glide the finger in carefully.

With the patient in the standing position, my finger can probe more deeply, and I can quickly tell if the right side of his gland feels exactly the same as the left. Of course, the most important part of the rectal examination is the search for any unusually firm, even rock-hard, surfaces that may indicate the presence of cancer. The standing position also allows me to complete the procedure in a matter of seconds—and the patient is usually happy about that.

I have yet to find a patient who enjoys this examination. Some patients joke about it—"Does your mother know what you do for a living?"

I am often asked how I could possibly remember the size of a patient's prostate from one year to the next when I must be doing thousands of examinations every year. My notes indicate my guess regarding the size of the gland and tell me whether it was soft, rubbery, firm, or irregular, or if it contained any other indicators that something might be wrong.

Patients also ask me how I can detect a tumor on the other side of the gland, when only the back surface can be felt by my examining finger. My response is quite simple: Seventy percent of all cancers originate in the area of the prostate that is easily accessible to me.

Cystoscopy

It's true to say, I think, that every man dreads the thought of a pencil-thick instrument being inserted into his penis and through to his bladder. Some men, so fearful of another cystoscopy, have been known to abandon follow-up care. Other patients have written about their ordeals.

I recall one disquieting yet entertaining article that appeared some years ago in *Esquire* magazine on this topic. Cystoscopies and vasectomies qualify as popular topics for masochistic confessions, but not always for good reason.

One of my patients, who has a bladder problem, has had six or seven cystoscopy examinations and tells me, "I don't mind the procedure at all because I know that it gets to the heart of the problem. If the urologist is as gentle as you are, it doesn't hurt much at all. It's a little uncomfortable when you move that thing around, but other than that it's not hard to take at all."

Actually, some urologists are considerably more gentle than others. I'd stay away from a urologist who says, "It's gonna hurt, so let's get it over with quickly."

A gentle urologist will ease the passage into the penis with a generous glob of lubricant that contains a mild local anesthetic called xylocaine. He or she will then insert the cystoscope slowly. As the instrument passes through the sphincter, which keeps the urine in the bladder, a little bit of short-lived discomfort is usually inevitable.

A nervous patient who cannot relax his muscles is likely to feel more pain than others. Sensation is also felt as the instrument passes through the prostatic urethra—the urinary passage through the prostate. There is only mild discomfort once the instrument is in the bladder.

Without removing the shaft from the patient's urethra, the urologist can insert lenses that allow him to inspect the bladder from various angles. A "zero" lens enables the doctor to look straight ahead, a "thirty-degree" lens allows him or her to look down thirty degrees, and with a "seventy-degree" lens he or she can examine at an angle of seventy degrees. By changing the lens, the urologist can inspect both the urinary passage and the bladder quite thoroughly.

Recently, the introduction of a flexible cystoscope means that the cystoscopy can be carried out without positioning the patient for childbirth (feet in stirrups). Finger controls allow the urologist to snake the instrument in the direction he or she desires, and since the instrument is smaller in caliber, it is less distressing to the patient. The field of vision the flexible cystoscope provides, however, is narrower, and this means that the examination might not be as thorough. So sometimes, the traditional instrument—which is a lot older than most practicing urologists themselves—can be a more exacting method.

A cystoscopy used to be a routine examination for prostate assessment. Today, we administer cystoscope examinations only to those patients whose prostate troubles are accompanied by blood in the urine. Cystoscopy may detect either a bladder tumor or bladder stones. By this method, we can examine the prostatic urethra to ascertain if there is any obstruction, or "kissing" lobes, for a distance of up to 2 inches (5 cm).

Prostate imaging

The prostate gland can be imaged indirectly, but somewhat incompletely, by a method called an "intravenous pyelogram." In this test, the patient, who has been prepared by a bowel clean-out (enema) and dehydration (nothing to eat or drink after midnight), is injected intravenously with a contrast material that contains iodine. The fluid shows up on an X-ray as if it were bone. The dye is excreted by the kidney and outlines it as well as the ureters and bladder.

The final X-ray is taken after the patient has emptied his bladder. The urine retained in the bladder is called "residual urine," and the X-ray image will show this and any indentation on the floor of the bladder that may be caused by an enlarged prostate gland.

A computerized tomogram scan (CT scan) depicts the body as if it had been guillotined at different levels, about half an inch (1 cm) apart. The test can be done with or without the injection of iodine. The cross-section image created by the computer reveals any lumps or bumps. The size and contour of the prostate can be seen during this procedure, but not the finer details that we would see with either a magnetic scan or an ultrasound.

The nuclear magnetic scan provides much the same type of

imaging, with more detail. It cannot, however, diagnose the presence or absence of cancer in the prostate.

Ultrasound imaging of the prostate gland, done with a cigar-shaped probe that is inserted into the rectum, was introduced by Dr. Hiroki Watanabe of Kyoto, Japan. His original equipment was crude, indeed. It was fixed to a chair and the patient was expected to actually impale himself upon it. The resulting image showed no more than bumps and lumps on the prostate's surface but was unable to detect any other irregularities within the gland itself.

Dr. Watanabe's early audiences laughed and said, "Well, maybe this will work in the Orient," implying that patients there were more stoic. His doubting colleagues did not believe that this was the beginning of a revolutionary advance in the assessment and examination of prostate problems—on a television screen.

The Japanese doctor's original equipment was crude in other ways. He probably used only a few sound waves and only those that were available at that time. Today, however, with machinery that can be adjusted by the flick of a small switch, a urologist can measure the density of a prostate gland with as many as 7.5 million sound-wave cycles per second. Interestingly, the human ear hears sound waves between 20 cycles and 20,000 cycles per second, while dogs can hear sounds of infinitely more than 20,000 cycles per second. The ultrasound waves "see" deep inside the gland. Sound waves bounce off fat, glandular tissue, muscle, and cancerous tissue quite differently, and the results can form telling images on the screen.

With this method, the prostate can be measured in length, width, and height, and by multiplying the three measurements by 0.52 (a mathematical factor designed for a prostate-like shape), a volume measurement of the gland can be obtained.

This is most useful in determining what kind of surgery a patient may need—incision or through the penis.

The gland itself is revealed on the television screen as a mottled gray organ, with the inner part clearly distinguishable from the outer part. Within the outer part there may be areas that look darker (hypoechoeic) or lighter (hyperechoeic). Again, this is of paramount use in detecting cancer, which is most often displayed as dark spots that may not be felt with the finger.

The PSA

Finally, we come to the blood test known as prostate-specific antigen, that protein which is secreted by every glandular prostate cell and whose function is to turn the gelatinous ejaculate matter into liquid. This simple blood test, which takes only a matter of seconds to perform and requires no dieting or special preparation, has become a marker for prostate cancer. This is because most prostate cancer cells produce ten times more PSA than noncancerous prostate cells.

Confusing the issue are two facts: PSA counts will be higher when there is prostate enlargement or prostate infection, and some cancers do not secrete the protein at all. Thus, an elevated PSA does not necessarily denote the presence of cancer.

The perfect prostate cancer marker would be a measurable chemical that is released only by cancer cells and not by normal ones. Alas, no such marker is available—yet.

Such are the ways to diagnose prostate problems. As the years roll on, there will doubtless be more. As society ages and our clinics and hospitals are called upon to treat more and more urinary dysfunctions, new ways to see or feel the geography of this troublesome little gland will be in even greater demand.

3. Enlarged prostate: The signs and the symptoms

Each year, urology clinics in virtually every major center throughout Canada and the United States are jam-packed with men who complain they cannot urinate properly. Usually, this is because they have what urologists call "benign prostatic hyperplasia"—a condition in which the prostate gland enlarges, or swells, and constricts the urethra.

The cause of this annoying problem can be manifold. Very often, though, it is simply because men have been taking any number of off-the-shelf medications for coughs and colds. They might have taken Sudafed, Robidrine, Benylin, Dristan, Sinutab, Novahistex, Robitussin, Actifed, or any other decongestant. Almost always they have neglected to read, or have ignored, the warnings on the package labels—that these medications should not be taken in the presence of symptoms of an enlarged prostate or any other urinary problem.

Understandably, then, some of my most grateful patients have been those for whom I have done nothing more than provide temporary relief from an enlarged prostate with the relatively simple passage of a catheter in their urethras—and a warning against all future use of decongestants.

It's worth mentioning here that one of the urologist's most valuable tools is a Foley catheter, so named because it was invented by an American doctor named Frederick E. B. Foley. It was first marketed as far back as 1934. Essentially, this is a two-channel length of flexible, hollow, rubber tubing that allows urine, blood, and irrigating fluid to continuously drain from the bladder.

One channel in the wall of the catheter connects to a small balloon that, when inflated inside the bladder with 10 milliliters of water, prevents this ingenious draining system from falling out.

The catheter—it comes with a urine bag that is strapped to the leg and must be emptied every three or four hours—is used to temporarily drain the bladder in cases when normal urination is impossible. It can be used more permanently for those patients who have lost control of their normal bladder functions. Many men wear a Foley catheter while having treatment for severely enlarged prostates and prostatitis, sometimes before prostate surgery, and always after it (temporarily).

Should the catheter plug with tissue or a blood clot, as is often the case in the early hours following surgery, manual irrigation is necessary. A little sterile water is pumped into the channel that drains the urine, and this is usually enough to ease the blockage.

What is an enlarged prostate, and how does it get that way?

As we have discussed, before puberty the prostate gland is a tiny structure that "sprouts" with the surge of the male hormone testosterone. By adulthood, it has grown to the size of a walnut. The prostate is a gland that exists only to secrete fluid.

To understand how and why it enlarges, however, we must consider its composition again: One-half consists of glandular cells, the other of a supporting framework that is composed largely of muscle cells and connective tissue. Imagine the prostate gland as a box of picked raspberries lying in a bed of straw. The berries are the gland, and the straw the muscle cells. In an enlarged prostate, there can be more or fewer berries as well as larger berries and/or more or less straw.

Generally speaking, when the enlargement is mostly glandular, or berrylike, the gland can grow to an enormous size without totally blocking the urinary stream. Overgrowth of the muscle cells, however, is likely to cause obstructive symptoms earlier. In many instances, the growth—or enlargement—is in both elements, which means that the urine flow is nearly always impaired.

It is easy to imagine how an enlarged prostate wrapped around the urinary passage can impede or block the flow of urine. The effect is similar to a kitchen sink that is slow to drain because debris is clinging to the walls of the pipe beneath it. In the same way, the urine spills slowly from the bladder when the passage is choked. Sometimes it is released in spurts, with stops along the way. Other times, the urine stream can be thin and require a lot of forcing.

But why does an enlarged prostate cause patients to void so often, with such urgency, and with such a frequent need as to interrupt sleep?

These irritative symptoms make sense if there is an associated urine infection, if there are stones in the bladder, or if the bladder does not completely empty out. Often, though, there are no such findings. All that is apparent is an enlarged gland, and a frequent and urgent need to pass perfectly clear urine, particularly during the night.

Is it because the neck of the bladder is being stretched by the prostate, triggering the need to urinate? It seems a logical explanation, but these same symptoms occur in older women, and they do not have prostate glands. Thus it is more likely the symptoms are from bladder irritation than from prostatic enlargement.

The bigger question is this: Why do so many prostate glands enlarge in middle age? The simple answer is that we don't really know. What we *do* know is that eunuchs—males who underwent prepubertal castration—did not suffer from enlarged prostates. In other words, all those male sopranos who were castrated as boys in the Middle Ages were spared visits to urologists! This is because castration eliminates the Leydid cells inside the testicles. Since these cells produce testosterone, there must be a causal link between an enlarged prostate and the presence of male hormones.

It is also true that this problem is more common in some parts of the world than in others, quite obviously implicating environmental factors and probably the different diets and lifestyles that come with them. We also know that when men emigrate from areas where an enlarged prostate is uncommon (like Japan) to areas where it is very common (like the United States) this geographical "protection" is lost within about twenty years.

The culprits are probably animal fats, which are believed to encourage prostate cancer, while the protective foods are thought to be soy products, which are believed to discourage it. Yet despite popular thinking among both patients and their partners, there appears to be no statistical link whatsoever between an enlarged prostate and prostate cancer. In other words, just because a man has an enlarged prostate does not by any stretch of the imagination mean that his gland is more likely to become cancerous.

To try to make this point—and to prove that environment

can be directly responsible for many causes of enlarged prostates—I have long lobbied for a study to be done on Caucasian men who have lived in Japan for more than twenty years. I would like to establish whether or not these men—like their native Japanese friends who live alongside them in the same cities and with access to the same food—are relatively immune, not only from an enlarged prostate, but from prostate cancer, too.

What we know more definitely is that, statistically, enlarged prostate problems are more common in certain families. Indeed, when they appear in men in their fifties, their brothers are four times more likely to require treatment for them, too. The reasons may be obvious: Family members tend to share the same diet and the same lifestyle, not to mention similar genes, which may be genetically responsible for the problem.

At present, the genetic basis for an enlarged prostate is still being investigated, but the results are not yet known. More certain within the medical fraternity is that cells in an enlarged prostate contain more growth factors and appear to live longer, thus giving rise to the possibility that an enlarged prostate may be passed from father to son.

If a genetic explanation for this common ailment is likely, the specific gene, or genes, have yet to be identified. If and when this happens, genetic engineering may well provide a cure for an enlarged prostate.

There was a time, about twenty years ago, when urologists deliberated very little before deciding how to treat a patient with an enlarged prostate. Nothing much was available to them. A patient who was complaining enough was encouraged to have the enlarged tissue carved out. So certain were urologists that the disease was progressive—that it would worsen and cause total urinary blockage—that even those patients who did not complain much were advised to submit to surgery.

Indeed, only in the last two decades has it become apparent that an enlarged prostate is not necessarily progressive and that its symptoms do not necessarily match prostate size. We now know that a man can have a prostate the size of a grapefruit and have no blockage at all, while another with a normal-sized gland might be unable to urinate, or be "in retention."

The term "prostatism," which once meant symptoms from an enlarged prostate, has been displaced by "lower urinary tract symptoms" (LUTS). The designation of a new term, however, added little new insight, but other things did.

Flow studies

As is so often the case, necessity has become the mother of invention. Thanks to the emergence of flow studies and ultrasound methods of measuring urinary retention, we now have greater insight into the correlation between prostate size and urine flow.

In a flow study, the patient voids into a special funnel instead of into a urinal, and the amount of urine passed per unit time is recorded on a graph. In a normal male, the peak flow rate should exceed 15 milliliters per second. When the peak flow rate is under 10 milliliters per second, it suggests prostatic obstruction—although a weakened bladder muscle or a stricture in the urethra can cause the same poor performance.

A pressure-flow study can distinguish a weak bladder muscle from a mechanical obstruction. In this test, the pressure generated within the bladder is measured along with the flow rate. If the flow rate is poor but the bladder pressure high, it suggests increased resistance, as from an enlarged prostate. If the flow is poor and the bladder pressure is low, the problem may not be related to prostatic obstruction at all. A bladder that has lost its muscle tone, because of diabetes, perhaps, or simply through having been overstretched during a long period of urine retention, also gives such a result.

Ultrasound residual measures the amount of urine left in the bladder after urination. In this method, a flashlight-like device is rubbed on the skin of the lower abdomen, generating a printout of an image that shows the amount of urine retention. Normally, there should be less than 50 milliliters of urine left behind in a bladder after urination. A residual of more than 100 milliliters is considered significant; residuals between 50 milliliters and 100 milliliters are in the gray zone and are subject to different interpretations.

The International Prostate Symptom Score

Test Name and Questions

The International Prostate Symptom Score (the IPSS) is a standardized questionnaire. From its battery of questions, seven stood up to statistical analysis. Three of these related to irritative symptoms:

- How often do you have to urinate within two hours of last having passed water?
- How often do you have an urgent desire to urinate that cannot be postponed?
- How many times must you urinate during the night?

There were then four questions that related to obstructive symptoms:

- How often do you have a weak stream?
- How often do you have to push to urinate?
- How often does the stream stop in mid-flow and need to be pushed to start again?
- How often do you feel you have not totally emptied your bladder?

The respondents' answers were scored from 1 to 5, depending upon the reported frequency of occurrence of the symptom during the past month:

Less than one in five times (1), less than half the time (2), half the time (3), more than half the time (4), and almost always (5). The scores were then added up.

I use this simple test often. Scores of 7 or less denote mild symptoms, and patients with these are best left untreated. Scores between 8 and 19 are considered moderate, and patients with these are good candidates for medical management. Scores between 20 and 35 are severe, and patients with these may require surgery.

Doctors, including urologists, are much too busy to have patients fill in their IPSS questionnaire in front of them. It may be given to patients to fill out while they are in the waiting room, or they may be asked to return with the form filled out on their next visit.

The symptom score is just a guideline. A patient with a high score may try his luck with medications, even though surgery has been advised, while another with a lower score may opt for surgery because he does not like taking pills for an indefinite period.

I find the IPSS useful because it helps me advise my patients. Some patients tell me that on another day, depending upon their mood, their scores might be different. Curiously, the symptom score does not include degree of urinary dribbling, which many patients find most annoying.

"No matter how long I stand there shaking it, a few drops are sure to stain my shorts," men typically complain.

I advise these patients to place their hand under and behind the scrotum, to lift up and massage the passage forward. The postvoid "dribble" can be lessened by this maneuver.

Such are the trials and tribulations of the enlarged prostate. Because of our aging society, and until new drugs are developed, our hospitals and clinics are likely to be inundated with men who cannot urinate properly.

4. Enlarged prostate: Medical treatment

Twenty years ago, before the advent of suitable drugs, there was only one treatment for an enlarged prostate—cut it out! And given that surgical techniques were not as plentiful and sophisticated then as they are today, this could be a painful ordeal. Now, there are many ways to solve problems caused by an enlarged prostate—and a wide variety of medications. Indeed, the choices have become bewildering, even to practicing urologists.

The prostate-shrinking pill

In the mid-1980s, when Merck Pharmaceutical developed a drug called Proscar (finasteride), which could actually shrink an enlarged prostate, it thought it had solved all enlargement problems. It was counting its bountiful windfall too optimistically.

The company knew that 20 to 25 percent of the income of all urologists came from carving channels in enlarged glands—a surgical procedure known as transurethral resection of the prostate (TURP), the most frequently performed operation in the United States and Canada after cataract extractions.

To address this dilemma, Merck carried out market research. It learned that between 55 and 60 percent of all men in North America develop prostate enlargement. Of this population, it discovered that only 3 percent had surgery, 17 percent consulted doctors, and an amazing 80 percent did not bother to seek any medical help whatsoever, certain that their urinary problems were just part of the aging process. Many older men fervently believed that nothing could be done for them anyway—or that if they consulted doctors they would be forced into an unwanted operation.

Actually, long before the Merck market survey, it was recognized that prostate enlargement started in most men after age forty, and was present in 50 percent of men in their fifties and 80 percent of men in their eighties. This was determined by pathologists. They had examined the prostates from men of all ages and determined that the disease starts as a nodule in the middle of the gland, in an inner area of the prostate known as the transitional zone. From there it grows by a little over half a gram annually (actually 0.6 g), gradually compressing the remaining normal prostate tissue, converting it into tissue like the pulp-peel of an orange.

The growth of prostate tissue may not be as regular as I have implied but may occur more in fits and spurts so that there may be long periods when there is no detectable progression in prostate size at all. Certainly, that is a pattern seen in clinical practice: A man may have an enlarged prostate causing minimal symptoms, and these may remain with him for years. Then, for no apparent reason, there may be symptomatic progression associated with an obvious increase in the size of the gland.

The story of how the Merck scientists created the pill to shrink the prostate has been told many times. A handful of men, possibly inbred, and living in the Dominican Republic, lacked an enzyme called "5-alpha reductase" from birth. This enzyme was responsible for converting testosterone into its more powerful form, dihydrotestosterone. When this conversion failed to occur, a boy was born with a sex organ that, even though it was external, made him look more like a girl. His penis was so small, it could be mistaken for a clitoris, his testicles were undescended, and his scrotum so scanty that it resembled labia.

Sometimes, the boys were raised as girls until, at puberty, they developed all the features of the adult male: a normal-sized penis, testicles in the scrotum, and a triangular-shaped patch of pubic hair pointing to the belly button. Inside the bodies of these adolescent males, however, the prostate gland did not enlarge.

"What if this enzyme activity were to be blocked in adult life by a simple pill?" the scientists wondered. "Would the prostate gland stop enlarging? Would enlarged prostate glands start shrinking? Could a pill make such a difference?"

Chemists at Merck, however, were not the only ones working toward restricting prostate enlargement. Scientists at Smithkline Beecham, Glaxo, and other pharmaceutical firms were also hard at work on a solution. Merck simply won the race, and in so doing many thousands of men across the world were able to see considerable improvements in their prostate woes.

How does the pill work? If testosterone is converted to dihydrotestosterone in the presence of the enzyme 5-alpha reductase, how can that enzyme be eliminated? Through a process known as competitive inhibition, that's how. If we make a molecule that has the chemical appearance of testosterone but doesn't behave like it, the enzyme 5-alpha reductase latches on to it, gets blotted up by it, so to speak, and is thus unavailable to make the conversion it was supposed to carry out—that is, from testosterone to dihydrotestosterone.

When Merck Pharmaceutical originally asked urologists at McGill University, among many other centers, to conduct Proscar's phase-three studies, the secret drug was called MK-907. The study was double-blind and placebo-controlled. This meant that neither the patient nor the doctor knew who was getting the pill that contained the active drug and who was getting the pill that looked the same but contained no active ingredient.

The drug trial showed that MK-907 did indeed shrink the prostate by about 20 percent, increase the maximum urine flow rate by 3 milliliters per second, and lower the PSA count by 40 percent in six months. The 20 percent shrinkage may not seem like much, but when it occurs where it counts it can be significant. The maximum flow rate change from 7 to 10 milliliters a second may be a difference of only 3 milliliters a second, but it can be the difference between discomfort and comfort.

It has been argued that the drop in the PSA reading (40 percent in six months and 50 percent in twelve months) can confuse the diagnosis of cancer, but the argument can be turned around. I have placed some patients on the Merck drug with the understanding that a biopsy would be undertaken if the anticipated PSA drop did not occur. Certainly, it is important to get a PSA reading before starting any patient on the pill.

In the trials, 1-, 5-, and 10-milligram doses were tried. There was little difference between the effects of 1 and 5 milligrams, and no difference between 5 milligrams and 10 milligrams. The company settled on marketing the 5-milligram daily dosage. (Subsequently, a 1-milligram pill has been put on the market to help bald men grow hair. This is called Propecia.)

Proscar had negative features, too. Five percent of those who took the pill suffered impotence that was reversed the moment they discarded the medication, and at least as many reported diminished erections. Ejaculate volumes dropped dramatically in all of these patients, and breast swelling occurred in a few. On the plus side, a number of bald men grew hair and some may have been protected from developing prostate cancer.

I recall Proscar being presented at a press conference when the pill was launched in Canada. "This pill may have the same impact Tagamet had on ulcers, eliminating 80 percent of surgery," I said. It was the clip used on television that night.

Although Proscar works well, with results that are maintained for several years, and continues to be prescribed, sales have not lived up to expectations. The pill shrinks very large glands—those over 40 grams—but does little for those men who have only slightly enlarged prostates. The smaller glands, however, tend to respond better to another family of drugs, called alpha-blockers.

The alpha-blocker story

If decongestants, or alpha-stimulation, can cause urinary retention, it seems reasonable to expect that alpha-blockers, with exactly the opposite action, can *improve* urinary flow, and they do.

Actually, alpha-blockers have long been on the market as good medications for lowering blood pressure. The pill achieves this by relaxing the muscle cells within the walls of the arteries. In much the same way, it reduces tension in the muscle cells within the prostate gland, thus helping many patients to void better and more comfortably. To those men who take them, and are happy with them, the effect is akin to a faucet that has been opened up to pass more fluid.

The first blood pressure pill in the alpha-blocker family that was used to help men with prostate enlargement was Minipress (prazosin), which was released in 1981. It worked quite well but had to be taken three times a day and was highly likely to cause a stuffy nose. Subsequently, in the late 1980s, Hytrin (terazosin) and Cardura (doxazosin) arrived on the scene. Both are to be taken in small doses at night and titrated to a higher effective dose. Five to 10 milligrams of Hytrin or 4 to 8 milligrams of Cardura are both widely used despite known side effects. Patients who sometimes complain of feeling faint or dizzy are cautioned to move slowly when arising from their beds, especially when they take the pill for the first time.

The latest medication in the alpha-blocker family is called Flomax (tamsulosin), which was approved for distribution in 1998. Unlike its predecessors, this drug more specifically targets muscle cells in the prostate, sphincter, and bladder neck and does not have as many side effects.

Flomax is promoted as a medication that does not require escalating dosages, or cause dizziness or fainting spells. In Japan, where this drug was developed, it is sold only as a 0.2-milligram capsule, rather than a 0.4-milligram pill as is the case in North America. This suggests that in Japan, where prostatic problems are less common, men can function quite well on smaller doses.

Although Flomax has become a very popular drug, some patients prefer the effects of Hytrin or Cardura, complaining that Flomax made them have a dry ejaculate (yet another side effect). Patients with increased blood pressure may be better off on Hytrin or Cardura anyway, and it will generally cost them less at the pharmacy. Unlike Proscar, the alpha-blockers work almost immediately.

Herbal preparations

Some people who promote food additives, herbs, and organic products have bamboozled the public into believing that, unlike the pharmaceutical industry, they have the citizens' best interests at heart. Unfortunately, exactly the opposite may hold true.

The pharmaceutical industry may be spectacularly profitable, but at least it operates under stringent government controls. Not so for food additives. Thus, products like saw palmetto are touted as every bit as good as Proscar with none of the side effects, with only anecdotal evidence and other testimonials as the basis for the claims.

I recommend saw palmetto in my practice because it is non-toxic, and a number of patients have been impressed with its effects on their urination. There is no study, however, that has demonstrated that—like Proscar—it can improve the urine flow by 3 milliliters a second, reduce the size of the prostate by 20 percent, and lower the PSA count by 40 percent in six months. Is saw palmetto better than the 30-percent improvement we can expect from a placebo product? I suspect it is, but I am not sure.

These remarks about saw palmetto—the best of the herbal preparations—may be applied to pumpkin seed (a good source of vitamin E, by the way), pygeum, stinging nettle, dwarf palm, rye, and several other natural substances that can be bought from health-food stores. I have to admit, however, that I have had no experience with these products.

5. Enlarged prostate: Surgical treatment

When all medications have failed, the urologist has no choice but to try to alleviate the symptoms of a large prostate with surgery. This, I am pleased to tell you, is relatively uncomplicated.

When I first started practicing medicine, the only operation for an enlarged prostate that I personally witnessed was a rather crude two-stage affair. In the first stage, a large rubber pipe about an inch (2.5 cm) in diameter was inserted, under local anesthetic, below the belly button and into the bladder. Two weeks later, the patient was wheeled back into the operating room, where, under a spinal or general anesthetic, the pipe was removed.

The surgeon then placed an index finger into the hole the pipe had left and, after breaking through the urethra, used it to actually gouge out the enlarged prostate tissue. When the index finger could not reach the prostate because the patient had a large belly, toothed forceps were used to tug the offending tissue free. Surprisingly, hardly any patients bled to death, although transfusions were more frequent in those days than they are today.

I suspect it was the prospect of having to undergo such an operation that kept many patients away from hospitals. It may also have been why so many men minimized their discomforts until they had developed urinary retention. Then they had no choice but to have this procedure.

Today, medical science has progressed beyond this. In fact, there are as many surgical procedures for an enlarged prostate as there are prostate-shrinking drugs; the choices have become bewildering. Furthermore, surgical treatments can be carried out either through the urethra or through the skin.

Some operations are minimally invasive procedures that rely on injections. Others are treatments that depend on the application of either heat or cold to eliminate excess prostate tissue. So, if you can't cut it out, you may be able to burn or even freeze it out!

Any major procedure in an operating room in any hospital requires the presence of a surgeon, an assistant (either a colleague doctor or a trainee urologist), an anesthesiologist, a scrub nurse, and a "floating" or circulating nurse. The surgeon is the acknowledged "star," but he or she can be upstaged accidentally, or deliberately, by the assistant, the anesthesiologist, or even the scrub nurse. It is not without reason that the operating room is commonly called the theater—and there can actually be some real-life drama there, too!

Before any kind of prostate surgery, the patient, often groggy from medications that are meant to sedate him and dry his throat, is wheeled from the ward to the operating room. Once there, he is placed on a specially designed table under the glare of overhead lamps.

The first specialist who sees him is the anesthesiologist, and I must tell you that medical treatment is never more intense than what he or she does. After all, it is the anesthesiologist that must ensure that the patient is completely prepared for the first incision. A lot of men I treat are petrified not so much about what I will do to them, but about how they will withstand whatever anesthesia will be used.

There are three kinds of anesthesia:

- spinal
- epidural
- general

The first two are regional, or local, anesthetics. For these, the patient must first sit on the side of the operating table, arching his back by bending over a pillow. This is to permit easier access to a space between the lower vertebrae, where the anesthesiologist's needle will be inserted.

In spinal anesthesia, a powerful drug is injected into the spinal cord itself. Once the spinal fluid has been located, the anesthesiologist is in the right place. The drug is administered. In epidural anesthesia, the anesthetist places a tube into a space outside the spinal cord. Here, with as many repeated doses of an anesthetic drug as necessary, he or she freezes the nerves.

When a general anesthetic is used, the patient is first put to sleep with a drug administered through an intravenous line that the anesthesiologist has inserted in his forearm. This takes effect within a matter of seconds. Then, a drug to paralyze all muscles is administered into the same line, and a tube is inserted into his windpipe to prevent him from swallowing his tongue.

It is through this endotracheal tube that the patient is ventilated and kept anesthetized with sleep-inducing gases, like ether or chloroform. In recent years, however, these agents have been replaced by newer, better, and safer drugs.

Blood pressure and heart beat are monitored continuously throughout all prostate surgery. In potentially complicated—and bloody—cases, a needle will be inserted into an artery in the wrist so that the patient's oxygen level in the arterial blood can be monitored. Another thin plastic tube may be inserted into the jugular vein so that the pressure in veins near the heart can be measured. This measurement helps the anesthesiologist decide if blood and fluid replacements during the operation are adequate, or whether they need to be increased.

While the anesthetic is being prepared, the circulating nurse ascertains that all the instruments and supplies are ready for the urologist to begin the operation. She wants to ensure that there are enough supplies, such as sutures, for example, and that all the instruments are in place. She also helps the scrub nurse keep an accurate count of the sponges, needles, and instruments used.

Like the surgeon, the scrub nurse is scrubbed, gowned, and gloved. It is the nurse's duty to pass various instruments to the surgeon as he or she works. A good scrub nurse will anticipate the surgeon's needs and have the appropriate instrument ready before he or she asks for it.

It is difficult to imagine operating-room procedure today without thinking of a lot of scrubbing of hands and arms, a lot of head coverings, gowns, boots, and gloves. Surgical gloves, however, were introduced only a century ago by Dr. William Halstead, a prominent American surgeon. He provided the first pair of these for a nurse suffering from a skin condition. Without them, she couldn't participate, and Dr. Halstead needed her help.

The operation starts with the surgeon, and/or the assistant, applying antiseptic paint like iodine to the area where the skin must be cut. Sterile drapes cover the patient from head to toe except for that part of his body that must be exposed.

Today, surgery is routinely required for extremely large prostates, that is, those over 100 grams. For this procedure,

I usually make a horizontal incision—"bikini cut," it's called—half an inch (1 cm) above the pubic bone. I then prize apart the recti muscles that run the length of the torso so I can view the frontal surface of the prostate gland. After that, I make a transverse cut over the prostate capsule, and, with my index finger, simply gouge out—or enucleate—the enlarged tissue. In other words, my finger finds the plane between the enlarged gland and the capsule formed by normal tissue that has been compressed by unwanted tissue. It's a bit like removing the fruit of a tangerine after the peel has been cut, and it is often just as easy.

This procedure, called a retropubic prostatectomy, was first introduced by the British surgeon Terrence Millan in 1947. The operation became established in the 1960s and remains a commonly performed procedure to this day.

Not long ago, in fact, I performed this operation on a sixty-four-year-old semiretired businessman who weighed 248 pounds (112 kg), stood 5 feet 10 inches tall (178 cm), and had denied, minimized, even ignored his health-care issues until he had passed a very bloody urine specimen. At this point he had had no choice but to consult his family doctor, who arranged an abdominal ultrasound examination. This revealed a solid lump measuring 2.1 inches (5.3 cm) long in his left kidney, an enlarged prostate gland, and four stones in his bladder, each the size of a robin's egg.

Any one of this man's three disorders could have been responsible for his bloody urine. A CT scan confirmed the presence of kidney cancer but showed no evidence that the disease had spread into the veins that carry blood out of the kidneys, or into the lymph nodes. A transrectal ultrasound assessment of the man's prostate gland, however, revealed it to be the size of a baseball, weighing 212 grams.

I proposed placing the patient on his side, removing his cancerous kidney, and then, if all was well, repositioning him on his back for a retropubic prostatectomy and the removal of the bladder stones through the same opening. I warned the patient that his excess weight put him at extra risk for wound infection, pneumonia, and phlebitis.

The three-in-one operation went smoothly, and his postoperative course was uneventful. The patient was so pleased with the outcome that he promised to submit to regular medical checkups in the future.

Consider, too, a sixty-six-year-old retired professor who, on rectal examination, displayed a very large, soft prostate, and clear urine that was nicely free of red and white blood cells. His very large gland and urine flow difficulties had suggested a need for immediate surgical correction, but this patient wanted to give a medical approach a longer trial. I agreed, recognizing that his woes were quite routine.

For one year, the retired professor had taken the alpha-blocker Cardura in 4-milligram doses, and Proscar in 5-milligram doses. His PSA count had now dropped from 12.0 to 5.8. An ultrasound examination showed that the prostate was calculated to weigh 140 grams, with no images that might suggest cancer. His improvement had been light, but, as he intended to travel extensively in the coming years, he finally took my advice and underwent a retropubic prostatectomy. Eighty-two grams of tissue was removed. Today, this man is pleased that he decided not to postpone the surgery any longer.

Transurethral Resection of the Prostate (TURP)

While the retropubic prostatectomy is a neat procedure with a predictable outcome, it has been challenged in popularity in recent years by what is called a TURP. This is the most com-

Transurethral Resection of the Prostate (TURP)

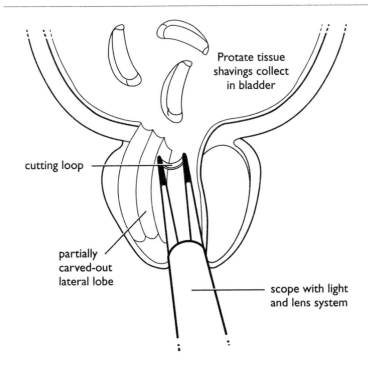

mon of all surgical procedures for an enlarged prostate. In fact, TURPs are now so popular among both doctors and their patients that, before useful medications were found, I used to perform several hundred of them annually, almost always with positive results.

The operation itself is really quite simple. After the anesthetic has been administered—either general or spinal—the patient, with his feet in stirrups, assumes the position of a woman about to deliver a baby. The genital area is then washed with an antiseptic solution, and the legs and lower abdomen are draped with a sterile covering.

The urethra is lubricated and dilated to accept a long metal pipe called a resectoscope (a variation of the cystoscope), which is about half an inch (1 cm) in diameter. It is fitted with a fiber-optic light that illuminates the passage and an electrical current powerful enough to function as a scalpel. The resecto-scope is passed through the tip of the penis and eased through the urethra into the bladder.

During the operation, the electrically activated wire loop is drawn back and forth rather like a crochet hook. With many short excursions of the loop—always from the farthest point to the nearest—the obstructing prostate tissue is neatly carved away. If arterial spurts are seen, as they often are, the bleed-ing can be stopped by switching the foot pedal, like a brake instead of an accelerator. This changes the nature of the cur-rent in the wire loop—from one that cuts to one that cauter-izes blood vessels.

When the resection has been completed, the tissue chips are flushed out of the bladder and a special Foley catheter is inserted to provide continuous irrigation. A smaller inflow channel allows a saline solution to wash out the bladder, and a larger outflow channel drains out the wash, which invari-ably contains some blood. When the drainage is largely blood-free, the inflow is stopped, and, within a day or so, the cath-eter is removed.

Patients usually urinate quite comfortably immediately after a TURP, though there can be some burning. The usual blood loss from the procedure is under 500 milliliters—a mere cup-ful—but about the same amount is lost after the operation as during it. Blood transfusions are sometimes necessary but are not routine.

Some measure of the surgeon's skill is reflected in the size of the prostate he decides to tackle, and sometimes pride over-rides prudence. A good urological surgeon can carve out 60 grams of obstructing tissue in less than an hour. Some experi-enced urologists can deal with a prostate that is not too severely enlarged within forty-five minutes. If the operation lasts two hours, however, it is usually far too long for comfort: Prolonged scratching by the resectoscope on the urinary lining can lead to scarring of the urethra. Such scarring causes a narrowing of the passage called a "stricture," and this may necessitate surgical correction in the future.

Today, TURPs can be performed with the surgeons watching their work on a television screen instead of looking directly through their resectoscope lenses. In this way, the operation can be done with higher magnification and without the surgeon having to contort his head and neck as he carves a passage through the tissue. Nevertheless, older urologists—generally used to employing the traditional method—feel more comfortable with what has worked so successfully for them for many years.

Whatever the method used, urologists aim to send all their patients home less than a week after their TURPs. It is a kind of success rate that comes with years of urological experience, and sometimes with inborn talent, too.

When things go wrong

The ideal TURP—60 grams of tissue pared away in sixty minutes—is not always achieved without complications. Sometimes, for instance, even when the surgeon feels he or she has limited bleeding during the operation, the patient may begin to lose a lot of blood in the recovery room.

Such was the case of a sixty-five-year-old schoolteacher who had had a routine TURP that went very well. When his bleeding worsened, I sought to slow it down simply by making the fluid that was irrigating the bladder—routinely at room temperature—ice cold. Fresh bleeding persisted, however. Clots formed within the bladder that could not be evacuated. Six hours after his TURP, the patient had to be taken back into the operating room.

There, copious clots in the bladder were evacuated with a syringe, but I could not discern where the bleeding had actually started. A rigid catheter known as a hematuric catheter that allows more vigorous irrigation was placed through the man's urethra into his bladder, and he was returned to the recovery room. There was no further bleeding, I am happy to recall, and the recovery proceeded normally.

What I have described here is not common, but not so unusual, either. Sometimes persistent bleeding during or after a TURP occurs because the irrigation solution was inadvertently allowed to run dry. The speed of irrigation is determined by the amount of bleeding; when bleeding is brisk, the irrigation must be rapid—almost a flow rather than a mere drip. Under these circumstances, a 3-liter (3 qt) irrigation bag can be used up quickly, and if it is not immediately replaced clots can fill the bladder.

Sometimes, the irrigation is as slow as an intravenous drip. Even then, if the nurse attending the patient does not replace an irrigation bag that has run dry, there can be problems with clot retention. Sometimes, a bleeding point has been insufficiently cauterized. At other times, an artery that has been in spasm, and had once appeared to be controlled, suddenly begins to bleed.

Such surgical setbacks can occur even when the patient is in the best of hands, but they are more frequent when a novice surgeon tackles too large a gland. Problems most often arise when the carving-out process has been too deep in some places—too aggressive near the bladder neck, for example, thus creating a nasty perforation—or too shallow in others.

When the resection is too shallow, the prostate tissue left behind falls into the cavity, obstructing the urinary passage, and there is no relief of symptoms. This can be corrected with a second procedure. Fortunately, unlike operations that require an incision, a previous TURP does not make a redo more difficult because there is no extra scar tissue en route.

When the cut is too deep, the prostate wall can be perforated. This may allow the irrigating fluid the surgeon has been using to accumulate in the tissue outside the urinary tract. At this point, the operation must be aborted because the abdomen will swell, and the patient will need a separate drainage procedure or time—usually a couple of days—to absorb the fluid naturally.

One patient who suffered this setback complained of severe pain—beyond the control of his spinal anesthetic—before the operation was completed. His abdomen began to swell enormously and became rigid. The procedure was halted and the bleeding was stopped by the insertion of a catheter—complete with a balloon that, when fully inflated, was able to plug the bleeding in the lower bladder. The man's intestines remained paralyzed for a few days but slowly recovered. No further surgery was necessary. The patient is grateful that he survived the ordeal and could urinate comfortably without more operations.

This second complication can be more critical. It is possible for unwanted irrigating fluid to actually enter large veins in the prostate area. This fluid contains a protein that simulates body fluid, but because it lacks salt, it will not conduct the electricity the surgeon needs for his resectoscope during the operation. When large amounts of this fluid are absorbed into the bloodstream, the sodium becomes depressed while the volume of water increases. The result is a form of water poisoning. The patient becomes confused, agitated, even temporarily blinded and comatose—a condition known as "TURP syndrome."

One such patient was a man of eighty-six. He had no medical history of serious health problems and, despite his age, was not considered a high-risk TURP candidate. The procedure was uneventful until it was almost complete. The man became agitated and nauseous, and retched. The anesthesiologist reported a rise in his blood pressure and asked me if he might be absorbing fluid.

It was possible, indeed. A few moments were taken to assure adequate control of all bleeding, and I terminated the operation immediately. Later, in the intensive care unit, the patient complained of blurred vision, then loss of vision. Usually, a patient in this condition must be treated promptly, with strong diuretics (water pills) and intravenous infusions of concentrated saline, or he may die. Fortunately, this one needed neither treatment. In fact, the statistics were on his side. While one in a hundred TURP patients may suffer this complication, few will succumb to it. In fact, in my entire career, I have never witnessed a TURP-syndrome fatality.

I have taught a generation of resident doctors how to do this operation, and it continues to fascinate me how some of them struggle endlessly to master it, while others do so with an economy of effort and style. I suspect it is like learning to accomplish reasonable heights in a sport. When it comes to manual dexterity and the perception of three-dimensional configurations, some people are simply more gifted than others. Both of these attributes are needed to restore a prostate to its normal function.

Side effects

A disconcerting side effect of the TURP is what is known as the "dry" ejaculation. There is ejaculation, in fact, except that the semen is now discharged into the bladder instead of externally. This is neither dangerous nor cause for alarm. It is a problem only to those patients who intend to father another child. In no way does it diminish the intensity of the orgasm. While many patients confess to being unhappy about the dry ejaculation, some actually revel in the fact that sex can now be "less messy."

More serious is the fact that 25 percent of patients who have had a TURP report diminished erections. Some say they have not been able to get an erection since surgery.

There is no good explanation for either of these conditions. Could the nerves have been damaged by the electrical current? This does not seem likely, unless the carving process was extended beyond the confines of the prostate. More certain is this: Patients are much more likely to blame the surgical assault for their erectile dysfunctions than to remember how imperfectly they may have performed before it. A much more likely explanation, then, is that the blood flow to the penis in older men is usually weaker than it once was—just as it may be somewhat diminished to the heart or brain.

Minimally invasive procedures

Complications with the TURP have encouraged a search for easier and simpler ways to manage enlarged prostate problems.

Balloon dilation may have been the first of the simple substitutes. A Foley catheter was adapted so that, upon filling its little balloon, it would distend the prostatic urethra that was obstructed by the enlarged gland. The idea was borrowed from the angioplasty for arteriosclerotic coronary arteries. The cholesterol plaques can be compressed like snowflakes, but prostatic tissue behaves more like shifting sand. Temporary relief lasting weeks, even up to a month or two, could be achieved by balloon dilation, but the results were much too short to justify the anesthetic involved. The procedure was abandoned.

A second, less-invasive method works very well for urethral strictures. It uses a scaffold-like contraption made of titanium, called a "stent." This is a short length of wire—like that used to contain chickens—that has been miniaturized and rolled into a cylindrical shape. When placed through a scarred urethra, the spring in the mesh distends the coil to a wider diameter, thus enlarging the opening. The titanium is inert to tissue reaction, and, within a matter of weeks, the "mesh" is overgrown by normal tissue.

The same coil can be placed through the prostatic urethra to keep the obstructing prostatic tissue from caving in. If the length of the coil is just right, it can work. If, however, the coil extends beyond the prostate gland, there can be problems. Stones may form on a section that reaches into the bladder, and a length that extends distally beyond the prostate will prevent the sphincter from functioning, rendering the patient incontinent.

With experience—on how to place this device accurately, and on how to improve its design—a role may be still found for the titanium-wall stent in the management of an enlarged prostate.

Thermal therapy

Heat and cold—and fire and ice—are not new. Government agencies, like the Food and Drug Administration in the United States or the Health Protection Branch in Canada, have no jurisdiction over medical devices that utilize extreme temperatures. Yet temperature has been part of our lives since time immemorial, and temperature is used to alleviate many prostate problems.

Without a government role, there are risks that hot/cold devices may be promoted with very little scientific validation. By the same token, however, honest efforts to invent and promote such devices may fail to get appropriate attention.

Devices that are used to raise the prostate temperature to 60 degrees Fahrenheit (16°C) do very little to the gland. Yet they are promoted to help people with prostatic symptoms. Just as a sauna makes a patient feel better, heat treatment may help his symptoms. There will, however, be no change in the size of his gland, nor an improvement in the flow of his urine.

Devices that raise the temperature of the prostate to 104 degrees Fahrenheit (40°C) are useful because they can destroy live prostate tissue, which leads to some sloughing and, consequently, a reduction in the gland's size. There may be a place for such treatment, but it is not appropriate for the severely enlarged prostate.

Another surgical way to treat an enlarged prostate is transurethral needle ablation (TUNA). This technique uses radio-frequency energy to punch holes in the prostate, lessening the resistance to urine flow. It is easily tolerated by patients. Its effectiveness, however, is less certain.

Whenever I suggest any kind of surgery, patients ask if I will use the laser. When I say no, they are invariably disappointed. They were hoping that a "magic wand" would be used.

"Would you use a blowtorch to light candles on a birthday cake?" I ask them.

When patients look at me as if to say "Why not?" I interject, "You wouldn't use a power saw to cut a matchstick, would you?"

Laser energy does have multiple uses in urological surgery, though. It has proven useful for superficial tumors of the bladder, for breaking up stones in the ureters, and for reducing prostate size by vaporization; that is, eliminating tissue that obstructs urine.

The first lasers for handling prostate enlargement shot beams into the prostate that had been reflected, by a mirror, at right angles. They killed tissue for varying depths and widths, depending upon the amount of energy used. The dead tissue was then sloughed and voided out over a period of several months. Dead tissue that was not washed out on urination, however, often obstructed the flow, and a catheter had to be left in place for several months at a time. Nonetheless, patients did not bleed, and for some this was a worthwhile treatment.

An example of such a patient could be someone on anticoagulation therapy, or one for whom temporary interruption of these blood thinners might be dangerous—a patient who has suffered a recent heart attack, for instance, and has been prescribed Coumadin.

Laser energy using holmium can also be used. It makes *direct* contact with the prostate and vaporizes tissue instantly. The holmium laser can carve out relatively large glands without any significant blood loss. In effect, it removes prostate tissue much the same way that my finger enucleated the gland in the retropubic prostatectomy. The laser tip finds the plane between the enlarged tissue and the compressed tissue that has formed the false capsule of the gland. The enucleated gland is then left to float freely inside the bladder.

At this point, another instrument, a morsellator, which can be likened to a meat grinder fitted with a vacuum cleaner, reduces the tissue to a pulp and sucks it out. That issue is then strained and submitted for pathological examination.

The holmium laser is an improvement over previous laser techniques and will find its place among all treatment options available.

These other options include:

- Microwave energy, which is also being used to ablate prostate tissue. This procedure is called transurethral microwave thermal therapy (TUMT). The microwave is generated by a device called a Prostatron, which is placed in the rectum. The heat it emits is captured by an antenna placed in the urethral catheter, and this heats the gland to a temperatures of between 40 and 167 degrees Fahrenheit

(64°C and 75°C), killing unwanted tissue, which sloughs out over a period of weeks.

- High-intensity focused ultrasound (HIFU), which involves ultrasound energy being focused precisely to produce comparable amounts of heat that can destroy prostate tissue.
- Cooling the gland to a temperature close to freezing, which can also destroy prostate tissue. This technique is being tried more to eradicate cancerous tissue than to eliminate unwanted tissue, but the principle remains much the same as that behind heat treatments.

You might think these different techniques represent totally different modalities of treatment. In fact, they just represent different ways of using hot and cold.

Cold can freeze the prostate and cause frozen tissue to be sloughed, but heat is generally more effective. Its use is akin to burning a hole through a block of wood by applying a red-hot branding iron to it, firing a blowtorch, or concentrating the rays of the sun with a magnifying glass.

Still another way to obliterate prostate tissue is by injecting chemicals directly into the gland. Pure alcohol can be used in this way, and it is both reasonably effective and very inexpensive. Promising results from this novel approach are just beginning to be reported. In the final analysis, however, an experienced surgeon can carve out obstructing tissue more completely, more precisely, and more effectively than any heat-generating and cold-generating devices available, although holmium laser experts may challenge me on this point.

Surgical studies

Surprisingly, worldwide urological studies done first in Denmark and later across the world throughout the 1970s and 1980s revealed that serious consequences, such as cardiac deaths in extreme cases, were more frequent with TURPs than they were with procedures that involved incisions.

How could this be? How could a procedure that eliminates a surgical incision, and therefore is considered less taxing on the body, be associated with such severe problems?

The urological community was shocked by these findings, and many centers began to reexamine their own results. Was it actually true that patients undergoing TURPs were more likely to have a cardiac death soon after surgery than those who had prostatectomies with an incision? And was it also correct that patients needed to return for second TURPs because of the regrowth of tissue more often than if they had undergone retropubic prostatectomies? By and large, these findings were confirmed.

At the University of Manitoba, a careful analysis carried out by Dr. Ernest Ramsey also supported these results. He reported that 13 percent of patients who had undergone a TURP required a repeat procedure. This finding compared with only 4 percent of those who had had an open prostatectomy.

Also, Dr. Ramsey maintained that the death rate among patients five years after TURPs was higher than among those who had undergone an open procedure. He discovered, however, that sicker patients were generally directed toward TURPs (rather than open procedures) because the former would be less traumatic for them. This meant that the deaths of these patients may not have been due to the effects of their TURPs at all, but from something else.

6. Enlarged prostate: The mimicking disorders

Many symptoms attributed to an enlarged prostate may not be due to this annoying condition at all. A scar in the urethra that has been caused by an infection—specifically gonorrhea—can create the same obstruction. Such scarring, however, is much more likely to be the result of an instrument having been passed through the urethra than of a sexually transmitted infection.

Urethral strictures are very often caused by simple catheterization, a routine procedure that can be damaging when it has not been done with adequate lubrication.

A stone in the bladder that is small enough to pass into the urethra will also impede urine flow and create a blockage that suggests an enlarged prostate.

Other mimicking symptoms are due to irritations rather than an obstruction. Patients who have these feel the same effects—the need to urinate frequently and urgently, both day and night. Diseases and disorders that create these annoying symptoms include Parkinson's disease, strokes, spinal stenosis, and multiple sclerosis.

Before telling you why prostate symptoms occur with these seemingly unrelated disorders, I would like to explain how the bladder works, and how urination normally occurs.

Make no mistake about it, the bladder is a marvel of engineering design, and when I lecture my medical students I talk about how this fine mechanism functions in normal life, and how it can be disturbed by different medical disorders. I usually start by telling them how the bladder gets short shrift in medical-school teaching because it is "a nonvital organ," one that is considered unnecessary for comfortable living—a kind of tank, if you like, that has been installed in the pelvic region simply to collect liquid waste. How unfair!

The kidney, on the other hand, receives a lot of time and attention because it appears to have a more important function. By producing large or small volumes of urine, the kidney is able to render the body either dry or moist. Also, by changing the acidity of the urine, it can make the body more acidic or more alkaline. In other words, the kidney is responsible for maintaining the body's healthy levels of acidity and liquidity while filtering unwanted fluid—urine—into the bladder.

Doctors like to manipulate, or fine-tune, the functions of the kidney by prescribing drugs like diuretics. These are "water pills" that essentially dry out the body by making a person produce more urine. On the other hand, doctors may advise a patient to add baking soda to a glass of water as an ongoing treatment for excess acidity. They may even tell a patient who has a history of kidney failure—uremia—to consume less protein so as to make fewer demands on the kidneys. Uremia occurs when the body cannot eliminate the end products of protein, and cannot control acidity or fluidity. This may lead to other distressing ailments.

Despite all of this, I can still tell my students that the work of the kidney can be done by a simple sheet of cellophane. They raise their eyebrows. Why? How?

A sheet of simple household cellophane is the essential component of the artificial kidney. As a semipermeable substance, it can actually strain the blood. As small molecules are able to pass through the pores of the cellophane membrane, the blood-fluid and bath-fluid equilibrate, and the waste products that have accumulated are washed out like dirt from clothing into the water in a washing machine.

You will see from this analogy that it is not too difficult to create an artificial kidney that can function outside the body for people on dialysis. To replace the bladder, though, would be next to impossible. The bladder, after all, requires a morass of nerve endings that tell us when it is time to urinate. Bladder muscles, on the other hand, enable us to actually do so—to enjoy this bodily function, naturally and fully.

If one of my lectures were a session with aspiring engineers, I tell my medical students, and I were to ask them to design a mechanical organ that had the properties of the human bladder, a mighty challenge would be in the offing. Engineers would need to create a receptacle that could hold liquid without it leaking, and yet, as it filled, develop absolutely no tension in its wall. Near its capacity the receptacle would also need to transmit a signal while still continuing to fill, now with a minimal increase in wall pressure. On command, the pressure in the wall of this receptacle would increase, causing it to contract and evacuate its content.

This, in essence, is how a healthy bladder functions. As it fills, it needs to have the properties of an ordinary plastic bag. Then, at capacity, it must transform itself into a muscular balloon that would literally thrust out the urine. If such a receptacle were made of plastic or metal, the task of urinating on the brain's command would be impossible. The engineers' "bladder" would have to have a faucet. By this reckoning, the human bladder operates as a miracle of anatomy.

How does it do its wonderful work?

The bladder muscles have a unique property that doctors call "accommodation." They use this word to define how muscle fibers in the bladder stretch, then relax automatically to accommodate an increased volume in urine without an increase in muscle tone.

When the bladder is almost full, there is a mild contraction of these same muscles that signals the sensation of fullness. The bladder muscles, however, can continue to stretch. Finally, upon voluntary command, they contract to evacuate the bladder's contents out through the prostate and the urethra.

This final contraction is rather like the knee-jerk reflex—stimulate the tendon below the kneecap with a rubber hammer and cause the leg to kick up as the quadriceps, or thigh muscles, contract. The reaction of the full bladder is like the tap below the kneecap, and the response to this is the contraction of the bladder muscles.

In a healthy person, this function is unconscious. It happens without a need to think. The bladder's reflex arc is connected to the brain by nerve fibers that travel freely up and down the spinal cord. Patients who suffer from Parkinson's disease, strokes, brain tumors, multiple sclerosis, and spinal stenosis, however, do not urinate quite so smoothly. These ailments destroy, disturb, damage, or blunt messages from the brain that normally tell the bladder *not* to contract. Without these proper "instructions," patients feel many more bladder contractions than normal—"uninhibited" contractions, as they are called in urology—often with nasty effects. In severe cases, the messages are so distorted that patients are unable to hold their urine at all.

This explains why patients who suffer from these ailments are often referred to urologists for prostate assessment when, in fact, they have no prostate disorders at all.

A patient suffering from congestive heart failure has a slightly different problem. His body will reabsorb the fluid that accumulates in his legs during the day, and this extra fluid, which has made his ankles swell, is voided out with greater-than-normal regularity. Again, the need to urinate often during the night has nothing to do with the prostate gland, but with an excess amount of water in the body.

Diabetes affects nerve endings at many levels. The sensation of bladder filling is less pronounced; consequently the bladder is often distended and rendered atonic—like an unburst but overstretched balloon.

Stones also cause extra irritation in the bladder wall, increasing the frequency and urgency to void.

Such reasons for disturbed urination patterns must be considered before assuming that prostate enlargement is the reason for the problem. Patients with the earliest symptoms of an enlarged prostate invariably complain of a frequent need to void in the morning—upon rising, for example, then ten minutes later, and again within an hour. After that, the urinary pattern becomes quite normal. How can I explain this? I can't. Not everything in medicine can be accounted for. I can, however, reassure patients that this is a common pattern.

Finally, a simple urine or bladder infection can cause the prostate to swell so badly that urination is impossible, sometimes for two or three days at a time. This condition is usually dealt with quite simply with any one of several antibiotics, including Septra (sulfamethoxazole-trimethoprim) and Cipro (ciprofloxacin).

But remember: No one should ever take a urine infection too lightly. It nearly always means that, for a variety of reasons that need to be accurately diagnosed, the prostate is not allowing the urine to pass freely. In other words, a urine infection could mean that the prostate is not functioning as it should.

Stay with me. We will now explore other symptoms that mimic an enlarged prostate as we discuss inflammation of the prostate and various other urological infections.

7. Enlarged prostate: Don't ignore your symptoms

If you are older than fifty, there is a good chance that enlarged prostate problems will affect your sense of well-being, particularly if they run in your family. For this reason alone, you should get both an annual rectal examination and a PSA blood test in a determined effort to ensure that, if your prostate is invaded by cancer, you and your doctor will know about it early.

Once the combination of the rectal examination and the PSA has ruled out cancer, the emphasis should be placed solely on dealing with enlargement issues. The important thing is this: Don't ignore any symptoms you may have.

When a patient chooses to overlook an enlarged prostate, his medical problems can move in several directions, almost all of them unpleasant indeed.

First, he can develop a sudden and total inability to empty his bladder—a condition known as acute urinary retention—one of the most painful ordeals a man can face. If he is catheterized promptly, and agrees to one of the several surgical options available, he should make a complete recovery. If, however, he is unfit for surgery—being within six months of a heart attack, for example, or having recently undergone a major operation—he might be temporarily helped by an in-dwelling Foley catheter that is changed every month or two.

On the other hand, his bladder might benefit from being drained via a catheter that is placed through his abdomen until such time as he can have corrective surgery. This procedure is called "suprapubic drainage" and, because the catheter does not traverse the length of the urethra and through the prostate, is generally considered safer for the patient because it avoids urethral strictures.

If I had to wear a catheter and a leg bag for a protracted period—more than two months, let's say—I would insist upon the suprapubic type. If I had a problem with incontinence, however, I might have no choice in the matter.

If a patient's urine retention is not immediately relieved, his bladder won't burst, but he will develop other problems. One of these will be the trickling of urine from the tip of his penis in what is called "overflow incontinence."

Should that same patient suffer a blow to the stomach during this time, his distended bladder could burst internally, spilling urine into his abdominal cavity and causing a severe infection, rather like a burst appendix. Without emergency intervention, the outcome could be fatal.

When the bladder cannot expel urine easily, it will first make changes to compensate for the increased resistance—a thickening of its wall. To put it simply, the overworked bladder muscles will thicken, just as biceps enlarge with weight-lifting exercises.

Following this, there is a process of decompensation—what we urologists call a "blowout" from the bladder wall. A distortion that resembles a sort of secondary bladder, this blowout is called a cellule when small and a diverticulum when large. The main problem is that a blowout, large or small, is not covered with a layer of muscle and does not therefore empty when the bladder evacuates. Thus, its remains indefinitely as a "bag" of urine, and, in some cases, stones will form within it.

The effects can be quite serious. Incomplete emptying of the bladder exposes the patient to many urinary infections, which brings us to another course a patient's health may take if he ignores treatment for his enlarged prostate—a gradual deterioration of his kidneys, a potentially more serious condition. Again, a thickening of the bladder muscles is responsible. This thickening can be seen when the attending urologist examines the bladder during a cystoscopy. The crisscrossing muscles that make up the substance of the bladder will give the lining a honeycombed appearance called "trabeculation." This causes a lengthening of the ureters, and these become tortuous and distended. More serious is that, where they actually enter the bladder, the ureters will be twisted into a fish-hook distortion that will cause the urine to back up.

Suffice it to say that patients who neglect to have these changes treated can eventually experience back-up pressure damage to their kidneys, for which the only treatment may be dialysis.

Monitoring your symptoms

My advice is to start keeping a record of your own symptom score—those lifestyle questions we call the IPSS—to see how they fluctuate, as they surely will. Consider IPSS readings as nothing more than a guide, however, and do not get alarmed if your score has increased over the years. This may be associated with the simple aging process.

Generally speaking, if your IPSS score is 7 or less, your urologist will probably decide to do nothing but monitor your condition lest it should worsen. If it is between 8 and 19 you may need medical treatment. If your score is 20 or higher you may need surgery.

Do not be shy about giving alpha-blockers a trial to help you urinate a little better—at any stage of your treatment or waiting period. It does not mean you will have to rely on them forever. If you tend to have high blood pressure, you might ask your doctor if you may try Cardura or Hytrin. If you have normal, or lower than normal, blood pressure, use Flomax.

When we stop and think about it, an enlarged prostate constitutes what I like to call a "plumbing problem" that must be fixed in order for the waste water to flow away. It is therefore wise to deal with it before it becomes a major issue that could affect kidney function.

It is debatable as to whether a change in diet or lifestyle can make any real difference to an ailing prostate once it has started to malfunction. This does not mean that diet couldn't have prevented the enlargement in the first place, although this has not been conclusively established. More certain is that a few diets and off-the-shelf medications have enjoyed some success in helping to alleviate prostate problems.

An innocuous herbal product called saw palmetto, which is derived from a small palmlike tree and is available in most health-food stores, has been known to diminish prostate-enlargement symptoms. I repeat, *only the symptoms* and not the enlargement itself have been affected. Saw palmetto has fewer side effects than Proscar because it is not nearly as powerful. Neither is it as effective.

It is worth my reminding you here that many off-the-shelf cold products have been known to aggravate prostate obstructions. I talk specifically, of course, about those decongestant remedies. If you catch a cold while you are experiencing voiding difficulties, it would be better to use Aspirin.

The prescription drug Proscar, meanwhile, is worthwhile if an ultrasound examination has determined that your prostate weighs more than 40 grams and is the cause of your symptoms. You should always ask your doctor for a PSA reading before starting Proscar so you will see your symptoms improve, and, consequently, your IPSS drop.

Many of my patients take both Proscar and alpha-blockers to promote urination. I usually start these men on the alpha-blockers and then add Proscar if the gland is well over 50 grams.

If your prostate is large enough—and annoying enough—don't be afraid of a TURP. In the hands of almost all surgeons, the results are excellent. Don't be afraid, either, of that inevitable side effect. Some men are actually quite grateful for internal ejaculation, particularly those who no longer want to father children!

Be prepared to listen to other options that may be more suitable for your particular circumstances than a TURP. If you are on anticoagulation medications, for instance, that holmium laser procedure is a very good choice for reducing a moderate-sized gland. If, however, your prostate is larger than 100 grams, consider the retropubic prostatectomy.

In the lifetime of an adult male there is more than a 50 percent chance of developing symptoms from an enlarging prostate. All the more reason, then, for you to view this problem as you would a receding hairline or the need for bifocals. Don't deny yourself the chance to live a full and enjoyable life. You may not be able to ejaculate as you did when you were younger, but your orgasms will be just as satisfying, and you'll be able to urinate so much more comfortably.

After surgery

Aspects of care following prostate surgery are fairly uniform, although the details may vary from hospital to hospital. At the Royal Victoria Hospital, the patient comes for a routine pre-operative assessment about two weeks before his operation. The resident doctor goes over his medical history, examines him fully, and arranges for an electrocardiogram, as well as the urine and blood tests, of which the PSA is only one. The resident will also consider a cross-match if there is a possibility that the patient may need a blood transfusion.

The anesthesiologist then arrives to discuss whether the patient should have a regional or a general anesthetic. Whatever the choice, the patient will be told to clean out his bowels with a powerful laxative the evening before surgery. Usually, he is admitted to hospital the day of his operation, having had nothing to eat or drink after midnight.

At the Royal Victoria Hospital, retropubic prostatectomies are carried out in a regular operating theater. TURPs, however, are done in a room designed especially for them. This is because each operation requires as much as 12 liters (13 qt) of irrigating fluid to flush out clotting blood and tissue. Regular operating rooms are not designed with the floor-drainage systems that can carry this waste away.

Whatever the procedure, the patient will have a catheter installed after his surgery. Pain-control medications are routinely prescribed, and blood tests are done again to check the degree of blood loss and levels of the natural blood ingredients.

A patient is discharged from hospital only when the urology team is satisfied that he can urinate freely after his catheter has been removed.

With minor variations, this is what to expect should you have surgery for prostate enlargement. You can avoid postoperative complications by breathing deeply even if it hurts, wriggling your toes and getting out of bed as often as you can to prevent inflammation of the leg veins (phlebitis), and taking no more painkillers than is absolutely necessary (these tend to make breathing more shallow and cause constipation).

Postsurgery constipation can be a menacing problem, and it is best alleviated with such bowel softeners as Colace (docusate), and by drinking lots of water that will also flush out the bladder and release blood clots.

Don't be alarmed if your urine suddenly looks bloody again. Following surgery, blood can remain in the urine for two or three weeks, even more. It does *not* imply another problem.

Finally, if you are cheerful, optimistic, and flexible, you will get better care and come out ahead.

8. Prostatitis: Bacterial

Of the three major maladies that afflict the prostate, the one most frequently misdiagnosed—and mistreated—is prostatitis, which can be either infectious or noninfectious, acute or chronic. It's worth mentioning here that 10 percent of all office visits to urologists, and 1 percent of all visits to family doctors, are prompted by prostatitis in various forms.

This whole area of prostate health, however, is not as clear as it could be, not only among general practitioners, but all too often among urologists as well. The result is that prostatitis caused by bacteria (an infection) is often mistaken for an equally debilitating form of prostatitis that is likely to be the result of a nonbacterial inflammation.

The problem is complicated further when we consider that nonbacterial prostatitis may have started as a bacterial disease, and that even though the infection itself may have been eliminated, it remains as an inflammation and continues to cause the patient a lot of pain and distress. Indeed, one problem often mimics the other, and the patient may simultaneously be suffering from both forms of prostatitis.

Broadly speaking, prostatitis simply means inflammation of the prostate—just as tonsillitis is inflammation of the tonsils, tendonitis is inflammation of a tendon, or pharyngitis is inflammation of the pharynx.

Acute bacterial prostatitis

Acute prostatitis is caused by a massive invasion of bacteria from the bowel, a condition quite easily diagnosed because the bacteria are isolated in blood, urine, or semen, or in all three. Thus, the urologist can examine any one of these components to reach a positive diagnosis. This is usually done after he or she has sent a blood or urine sample to a laboratory for analysis.

Some years ago, a Danish bacteriologist named Hans Christian Joachim Gram (1853–1938) discovered that all bacteria could be identified by adding a dye that turns them either red or blue. Doctors have used this system widely, and the term "Gram-positive" has come to denote one strain of bacterium while "Gram-negative" defines another. It is the Gram-negative bacteria—those that stain blue in the laboratory—that are the usual cause of bacterial prostatitis.

Other organisms, such as viruses, tubercle bacilli (the bacteria that cause tuberculosis), or those associated with sexually transmitted organisms like chlamydia or gonorrhea, do not usually cause prostatitis, although tuberculous prostatitis and chlamydial prostatitis have, on very rare occasions, been discovered.

How the bowel bacteria actually enter the prostate gland—whether in the bloodstream (via the venous system through the urethra), by traveling down the urinary tract from the kidney or the bladder, or by direct extension through the bowel wall—has not been positively ascertained.

Can bacteria from a bad tooth enter the bloodstream and settle in the prostate? Can an infected toenail resulting in a huge and swollen lymph node in the groin create the route? Can diverticulitis—an infection within a blowout in the intestine—lead to a direct invasion of bacteria into the prostate from the bowel?

The route of prostate infection may not be known, but the clinical manifestations of such a bacterial assault are clear. The patient suddenly falls sick with a high temperature and chills. He may need to urinate too frequently, experience painful urination, or be unable to postpone urination. In some cases, he may not be able to urinate at all.

How is acute bacterial prostatitis diagnosed? When I place my gloved finger in the rectum of a patient, my suspicions are confirmed when I encounter a hot and spongy prostate gland. I must remember not to carry out a vigorous rectal examination, though. Inadvertently massaging the gland might force a large amount of bacteria into the bloodstream, causing more serious problems that are immediately demonstrated by a high fever (septicemia) that can lead to a collapse of the cardiovascular system. This is the direct result of bacterial products called "endotoxins" in the bloodstream and has a 25 percent fatality rate without prompt and aggressive treatment. It is a condition not unlike the bacterial invasion we know as "flesh-eating disease."

Even without a rectal examination, a blood culture is always positive since a small amount of bacteria will have invariably found its way into the bloodstream. It is always discovered in a urine sample, too. The most likely delinquent organisms are e-coli, followed (in frequency of occurrence) by proteus, klebsiella, enterobacter, pseudomonas, and serratia.

Before a patient's culture results come back to my attention, I have already started his treatment for prostatitis with intravenous antibiotics. How can I possibly prescribe antibiotics without the benefit of laboratory results? The answer is quite simple. The condition is usually serious enough to warrant a judgment call—and a quick one; I prescribe antibiotics based on my experience of having treated similar cases in the past. The point is that some kind of treatment *must* begin immediately or else there may be a high price to pay.

Almost without exception, I am happy to say, my choice of medications turns out to be correct. Gentamicin (between 1 g and 2 g daily intravenously) and ampicillin (2 g four times daily) are the usual first-line drugs for acute bacterial prostatitis. They are administered together.

When these cannot be used because of an allergy, perhaps, or when the patient's kidneys are functioning poorly, quinoline antibiotics like Cipro (200 mg to 400 mg every twelve hours intravenously) are in order. Gentamicin is kidney toxic and should not be the first choice.

Sometimes I might prescribe a drug like Kefzol (cefazol) at the rate of 1 gram intravenously every eight hours. The clinical response is almost always prompt and dramatic, and when the patient is well enough, he is switched to oral antibiotics for a few extra weeks. Almost all patients are cured by these medications.

If a patient does not respond promptly to antibiotics and continues to have a spiking temperature (normal in the morning and rising to 103 degrees Fahrenheit [39°C] in the afternoon), I worry about an abscess in the prostate.

As in the case of an abscess anywhere else in the body, a prostate abscess must be drained. This is best accomplished through the urethra in a procedure not unlike the TURP. The procedure will require an anesthetic and a few excursions with a resectoscope. We know the abscess is draining when we see pus oozing from the incised prostate.

The urgent necessity of this procedure is best illustrated by recalling another of my patients—a forty-seven-year-old auto mechanic who came to the emergency room at my hospital in dire distress. He was flushed with fever, had a racing heart beat, and could barely pass water. The attending physician diagnosed an acute urinary-tract infection, and, after routine urine and blood cultures had been rushed off to the laboratory, the patient was immediately given antibiotics.

After he had been admitted to a medical ward for observation, the man seemed to improve. Later, however, he developed urinary retention and a urology resident was called in to install an indwelling Foley catheter. At this point, after detecting a red-hot prostate on rectal examination, the resident diagnosed acute prostatitis.

Over the next ten days the patient's dangerously high afternoon temperature spikes did not abate. A prostatic abscess was discovered, and a resectoscopic drainage of the prostate was carried out. The results were dramatic. As soon as pus oozed from his incised prostate, the patient's high temperature disappeared. From then on, his recovery was swift and smooth.

Chronic bacterial prostatitis

This chronic form of prostatitis is much more enigmatic. Three clinical types are recognized: chronic bacterial prostatitis, chronic nonbacterial prostatitis, and prostatodynia—chronic pain that emanates from the prostatic area, or is presumed to do so.

I see a number of patients who have been treated with antibiotics regardless of their conditions. Many have come to me for a second opinion because the pills haven't done them any good. When I ask them if the medications were prescribed following urine cultures, they often tell me that no urine sample was taken. When I want to know if a prostatic massage was carried out as a diagnostic measure, the answer is again negative. The pills were prescribed, I am left to conclude, on the basis of the patients' stories and their doctors' guesses.

I also see patients who have been dismissed by their doctors as whiners—those with low thresholds for pain and discomfort—when, according to my assessment, they do indeed have chronic bacterial prostatitis.

Chronic bacterial prostatitis is the diagnosis made most frequently with inadequate diagnostic criteria, sometimes correctly and other times not. Typically, the patient will be a young to middle-aged man who is sexually active and who has a history of previous urinary-tract infections. His complaints will include fatigue and malaise, low back pain, irritation or pain on urination (dysuria), and a much-too-frequent need to urinate both day and night. He will also have an itchy urethra while urinating, pain or discomfort when sitting, pain during ejaculation or after it, a loss of sexual desire, the loss of an erection, emotional distress, and even depression.

It may surprise you to know that a diagnosis of chronic bacterial prostatitis is quite often made purely on the basis of symptoms that later turn out to be psychological—symptoms based entirely on what a patient says about himself and how he describes his problem. Many of these cases involve men who have guilty consciences for having committed sexual indiscretions or who are suffering from valid clinical depression.

Recently, urologists have devised a system—not yet fully accepted by the specialty at large—to try to ascertain if symptom scores like the IPSS could help differentiate between prostatitis that is real and prostatitis that is purely psychological.

The system isn't perfect, of course. That's why respectable urologists, under the pressure of unending work, have been known to prescribe drugs for patients who do not have prostatitis at all, but merely some of the peripheral symptoms. We know, of course, that if a man has blood in his urine, and a combination of other blatant symptoms, he certainly has the disease. What we need to ascertain now, however, is what to do when a man displays only some of the less severe symptoms that might, on close examination, be attributed to something else.

Suffice it to say, then, that it is impossible to base a treatment for chronic bacterial prostatitis solely on a patient's complaints—especially when that treatment might involve surgery. One man I recall, a thirty-four-year-old graduate student, had this exact dilemma. His urologist was treating him for erectile dysfunction and, when all treatments proved unsuccessful, had suggested installing a penile prosthesis.

Understandably, the patient was in a terrible panic when he came to see me. He was indeed impotent, but more to the point, he had become so preoccupied with his inability to have an erection that he had minimized his other symptoms.

The fluid I obtained from this patient by prostatic massage showed that he suffered from classic chronic bacterial prostatitis, which turned out to be the source of his erectile dysfunction. I am happy to report that I was able to eradicate the man's prostatitis with antimicrobial therapy. His potency returned within a matter of days.

The point is this: It is really impossible to make a diagnosis on the basis of a man's complaints—that it is painful to sit, that his penis hurts, that his prostate feels tender when he ejaculates. An examination must be done to ascertain whether or not there are more telling signs and symptoms.

Diagnosis

The most time-honored method for diagnosing chronic bacterial prostatitis is a quantitative urine culture done before and after prostatic massage. Bacterial counts should be ten times higher in the urine specimen obtained after prostatic massage than in the first one, called a midstream sample.

Although this test was first reported by Americans Dr. Edwin Meares and Dr. Thomas Stamey in 1968, and remains the "gold standard," it is seldom done. A Canadian expert, Dr. Curtis Nickel, at Queen's University, in Kingston, Ontario, has suggested why. The test is enormously time-consuming and the monetary reward for establishing the correct diagnosis is disproportionate to the effort involved.

It takes at least half an hour to collect the urine sample, carry out a prostatic massage, and collect a second sample. According to government-run medicare schemes, the monetary reward for correctly diagnosing chronic bacterial prostatitis is a fraction of the reward for seeing three patients in the same time frame and making an incorrect diagnosis in all three. Furthermore, patients cannot always void on command after prostatic massage. Thus, most clinicians resort to the examination of the prostatic fluid after massage, looking for the presence of leukocytes (white blood cells) and macrophages that contain fat (oval fat bodies) under the microscope.

When there are fewer than fifteen white blood cells per high-power field at forty times magnification, the test is negative. When there are fifteen or more cells, often in clumps, the test is positive.

The massage should not be done within forty-eight hours after the patient has ejaculated. Prostatic massage taken within this time frame may show spuriously high leukocyte readings or may not yield enough fluid for examination.

Although the presence of leukocytes is not synonymous with the presence of bacteria, it is nonetheless a marker—and better than guesswork.

I once spoke to a gathering of primary-care physicians and suggested that microscopy should be mandatory in the absence of sequential urine cultures to diagnose chronic bacterial prostatitis. A doctor in the audience rightfully pointed out that microscopes were not part of the paraphernalia in a normal primary-care practice.

I began testing prostatic massage secretion on the leukocyte band of a dipstick and compared it to examination under the microscope at forty times magnification. I can now say that the dipstick can be used as a good substitute for microscopy. A dark purple, or a two-plus, reading corresponds to fifteen or more leukocytes per high-power field. If the dipstick contains a nitrite band, it is even possible to distinguish bacterial prostatitis from nonbacterial prostatitis. The nitrite band becomes positive when bacteria are present, not when leukocytes are present on their own.

Once the diagnosis of chronic bacterial prostatitis is established, antimicrobial therapy begins. I use Floxin (ofloxacin) and the trimethoprim-sulfamethoxazole combination of Septra or Bactrim (commonly sold as a double strength tablet containing 160 mg of trimethoprim and 800 mg of sulfamethoxazole), alternating the two drugs every two weeks for a minimum treatment of twelve weeks. After that, I often ask patients to take half the dosage—300 milligrams of Floxin daily instead of twice a day, or Septra one double strength instead of two, for a month—halving it further every month until only half a pill is taken each day for up to a year. When patients relapse, the dosage is raised to the starting dose.

In addition to prescribing antimicrobial drugs, I advise patients to cut out alcohol, coffee, and spices; to ejaculate frequently; and to bring heat to the prostatic area by taking hot baths or sitz baths. Most patients respond, but the problem often recurs.

The choice of Floxin and Septra or Bactrim deserves amplification. Floxin is one of the quinoline antibiotics, like Cipro (ciprofloxacin) and Noroxin (norfloxacin). Cipro is probably the most widely used quinoline today. It is well tolerated and very effective for most Gram-negative bacterial invasions of the body. Noroxin is well tolerated, too, and remains the best "strong" pill for the routine urinary infection.

Getting antibiotics into the prostate is so difficult that clinicians will favor drugs—like Floxin, which diffuses better into the prostate tissue—that have even a slight advantage. Recently, a minor modification of Floxin has resulted in a new drug called Levoquin (levfloxin). As this is a 500-milligram once-a-day pill, it will be favored over the twice-a-day dosage of Floxin. I have prescribed it in place of Floxin, but I do not know if it is any better. What I do know is that most patients prefer taking medications once a day rather than twice.

Septra was developed in the Burroughs Wellcome laboratories headed by the late Dr. George Hitchings. In one of my medical-student talks, I extolled Hitchings's genius. Here was a man, outside academia, who had a major impact on the practice of medicine. His team developed Zyloprim (allopurinol), which has forever altered the management of gout and uric acid elevation, and he introduced rejection-fighting Imuran (azathioprine), which launched the possibility of organ transplantation. He then introduced Septra, which was a combination of trimethoprim and sulfamethoxazole.

Here, however, I think he might have made a multibillion-dollar blunder. There is nothing wrong with this combination drug, but trimethoprim could have been combined with another sulphonamide rather than Hoffmann La Roche's patent-protected sulfamethoxazole.

If a trimethoprim-sulphadiazine combination had been released first, Burroughs Wellcome would not have had to share the initial profits with Hoffmann La Roche. The combination would have worked just as well and the company coffers might have been enhanced by billions of dollars. Clever people do make colossal miscalculations.

Perhaps there is another side to this story. Maybe the best results in the Burroughs Wellcome laboratories occurred with the combination of trimethoprim and sulfamethoxazole over trimethoprim and sulphadiazine. Rather than release an inferior product the folks at Burroughs Wellcome favored science over profit. I will stick to my story, though. The trimethoprim-sulphadiazine combination constitutes a product that is just as good in terms of bacterial coverage and effectiveness, has no increased side effects, and is a smaller pill that is easy to swallow.

I treat my patients with chronic bacterial prostatitis for twelve weeks on the full dosage of quinolones (Floxin or Levoquin) or the sulphonamide-trimethoprim combination, and for an even longer time on reduced dosages.

If prolonged antibacterial therapy has any merit at all it must be because indolent bacteria hiding within the prostate are difficult to eradicate. It makes sense, then, to heat the prostate to temperatures that can kill bacteria without causing excessive tissue injury—to about 104 degrees Fahrenheit (40°C).

It is just such a rationale that is behind hyperthermia treatment of the prostate, which we have already discussed. The machine used to treat enlarged prostates has also been tried on patients with prostatitis. Investigators in Israel and Italy have explored the use of hyperthermia to treat prostatitis, and some encouraging results have been reported—so much so that I have sent some of my own patients for hyperthermia treatment. The treatment is available in Canada but is not usually covered by medicare schemes.

Almost all patients report some improvement with hyperthermia treatment, but I do not know if they are merely trying to rationalize the money they have spent to have it, or if the heat may have dulled their pain by killing nerve endings. I would like to think that the treatment also killed bacteria.

The terrible consequences of severe bacterial prostatitis are probably best illustrated by another patient—a fifty-eight-year-old family practitioner, no less, who displayed all the symptoms associated with this chronic disease. He had read the first edition of my book *Private Parts* and felt I was describing him when I wrote about "symptoms that may combine to make life seem not worth living."

The physician asked me to take him on as a patient, and I agreed. I persuaded him to try all the different medications available for bacterial prostatitis, as well as hyperthermia.

When hyperthermia failed, the patient persuaded me to surgically remove as much of the offending prostate tissue as I could. I agreed to do this in a procedure I likened to a drastic TURP. Alas, this brought only brief and temporary relief.

Finally, the patient and I agreed on a much more drastic solution—the radical removal of his prostate, a procedure usually reserved only for cancer.

Fortunately, the outcome was successful and the patient has never regretted taking this step. I had warned him that the operation could render him impotent or incontinent or both. Chronic bacterial prostatitis had left him with an infection so deep and painful that he was willing to take the chance.

9. Prostatitis: Nonbacterial

The symptoms of nonbacterial prostatitis are almost indistinguishable from those of chronic bacterial prostatitis, but there is no infection. In other words, nonbacterial prostatitis is really inflammation of the prostate, and this causes the same kind of irritation we would expect when bacteria is present.

Was bacteria present originally but eliminated by antibiotics? Is bacteria present but undetectable, hiding under a biofilm (a thin protein layer, like veneer on plywood)? Or was bacteria absent from the outset?

The answers to these questions are not always forthcoming. Perhaps some cases of chronic nonbacterial prostatitis are originally due to bacteria. Others may have been caused by a urine backflow into the prostatic ducts, causing an inflammatory reaction not unlike reflux nephropathy.

In reflux nephropathy, which is largely a disorder that affects preschool children, urine is regurgitated from the bladder into the kidney tissue, where it initiates an inflammation that can scar a kidney. Severely damaged, shrunken, almost nonfunctioning kidneys have been the result of severe cases of childhood reflux nephropathy.

Experiments that use a catheter to fill the bladder with water containing Indian ink show that urine can, under a certain set of circumstances, penetrate the prostatic ducts. This investigative test was carried out a few years ago when a handful of patients, each about to undergo a TURP for an enlarged prostate, volunteered to have Indian ink instilled into their bladders via a Foley catheter three days before their operations. Doctors discovered that prostatic ducts in the carved-out prostate tissue contained the ink much more often in those patients with a known history of chronic nonbacterial prostatitis than in those without. This means that the regurgitation of urine into the prostatic ducts may well be the way in which chronic nonbacterial prostatitis occurs.

Whatever natural course the disease may have taken, I usually treat my nonbacterial prostatitis patients with the same course of antimicrobial drugs (Septra or Floxin, for example) that I would use if bacteria were present. I do this on the simple presumption that the problem might have a bacterial component. If patients respond to this—and many do—I continue the treatment as if their problems were bacterial, even though they might be otherwise.

If there is no response at all, I stop this treatment and substitute the antibiotics with nonsteroidal anti-inflammatory drugs. These include either Indocid (indomethacin), or Naprosyn (naproxen), or the newly released cox-2 inhibitors like Vioxx (rofercoxib) or Celebrex (celecoxib). Sometimes I add a muscle relaxant such as Valium (diazepam). I may also try Prosta (quercetin), a bioflavonoid dietary supplement that was recently found effective in a scientific study.

When pain is a major factor, I add a nighttime dosage of 5 milligrams of Elavil (amytriptylline), building up to a dosage of 25 milligrams. While patients are not always rendered pain-free with this treatment, many say it helps. A few patients, however, need to be referred to a pain clinic.

Sometimes I have to refer a patient to a psychologist or a psychiatrist because I feel he is harboring an underlying problem that I, as a urologist, am just not equipped to handle.

Consider the man who did the rounds of Montreal dentists, asking for them to remove his teeth because, he said, they ached incessantly. Eventually, after several extractions, he met a dentist who told him that his problem was in his head and not his mouth. He needed a psychiatrist because his pain was psychosomatic.

Such was the case of a fifty-two-year-old man who, when referred to me by his family doctor, was miserable with low back pain. He also had pain in his prostate area, pain in his upper thighs, pain on urination, pain on ejaculation, pain in his groin, pain in his lower abdomen, pain everywhere. The only positive finding was the presence of numerous leukocytes in fluid obtained after performing a prostatic massage.

Antibiotics did not help him, which suggested that there was no infection. Anti-inflammatory drugs, such as Naprosyn and Indocid, were ineffective, as were painkillers like Codeine and Percocet. Some relief, however, was obtained by combining Valium, Elavil, and the antidepressant Prozac (fluoxetine), but the patient's symptoms were still far from being controlled.

At present, he is coping with his discomfort, though he has virtually no sex life and must often be absent from work. In the future, he knows he may well need to seek help not only from a specialist in pain control, but from a psychiatrist as well. I believe that his discomfort, as severe as it is, is largely stress-related.

Prostatodynia

Although the pain associated with prostatodynia is in the area of the prostate, it has nothing to do with the gland itself. Urine cultures done before and after prostate massage are always bacteria-free, and leukocytes are invariably absent from prostatic secretion. The problem is presumed to originate from disorders of the muscles in the pelvic floor. Geographically, then, it appears to be the domain of the urologist when, in fact, it is really not urological at all.

Nonetheless, I treat it. A strong nonsteroidal anti-inflammatory drug, like Toradol (ketorolac tromethamine), may help some patients, and I often try this medication before all others.

If the patient's urine flow is poor, I prescribe Flomax, Cardura, or Hytrin. Treatment for prostatodynia with Elmiron (pentosan polysulfate), a drug for a bladder condition known as interstitial cystitis, is new, and I cannot yet comment on its effectiveness. I can, however, offer some comments on the condition itself.

Interstitial cystitis is a predominantly female ailment with many unknowns. No one knows, for example, what causes it, how best to diagnose it, nor even the most reliable way to treat it. Urologists are also baffled as to why it affects women 90 percent of the time.

What we *do* know, however, is that this aggravating condition is linked to the absence of a fine, protective layer of protein called glycos-amino-glycan (GAG), which lines the inner surface of the bladder to prevent urine from seeping into the bladder walls. In a healthy adult, that layer is there. Just as the protective coating of Teflon prevents food from sticking to a frying pan, the GAG makes the surface of the bladder less sticky to bacteria, and blocks urine from seeping first into the lining and then into underlying layers of muscle.

In interstitial cystitis, much of this GAG is lost, and urine is able to seep into bladder muscles, creating a nasty inflammation. This, in turn, causes severe pain, particularly as the bladder fills up. It lessens as the bladder is emptied but starts up again as the cycle is repeated.

Because the severe pain of this condition mimics that of nonbacterial prostatitis, or prostatodynia, Elmiron is being explored as a possible medication. Time will tell whether or not it will work.

10. Prostatitis: The last word

The more I think about it, the more I realize that I wouldn't wish prostatitis—acute or chronic, bacterial or nonbacterial—on anyone. It is all too often a diabolical disorder, debilitating and depressing, that has a man agonizing for days on end until his medications finally kick in. Sometimes medications don't kick in at all, and the patient is left wondering whether he'll ever urinate or ejaculate without pain again.

In truth, urologists don't much like treating this condition because good, lasting results take a lot of time, if they occur at all. They would much rather deal with a tumor or a kidney stone because these and similar conditions enable them to see the results of their work relatively quickly.

Should you be unfortunate enough to become afflicted with prostatitis, there are a number of safeguards to remember. First, you should insist upon all the necessary diagnostic measures we have discussed. Antimicrobial therapy should err on the side of overtreatment rather than undertreatment. Anti-inflammatory medications, muscle relaxants, painkillers, and other drugs can only be assessed on a trial-and-error basis.

There is no controversy about how to diagnose and treat bacterial prostatitis, either acute or chronic. Nonbacterial prostatitis and prostatodynia are, of course, far different matters. Because there are no specific diagnostic criteria for these—nor established treatments, for that matter—they are mysterious entities, indeed, and consequently lend themselves to all manner of witchcraft and quackery.

Much of this morass of deception, intentional or otherwise, is perpetrated on the Internet. Here, information is disseminated at will without peer-reviewed or editorial scrutiny. A person need only be able to type, after all, to have access to the Internet, either to gather information or to post it.

Of course, there is nothing wrong with a person lamenting his misfortunes on the Internet. Patients can, almost anonymously, spill out their hearts on the most private of matters. They may describe their battles with what they think is prostatitis, for instance, and tell how every expert urologist has failed them. Conversely, they often describe "successful" experiences with alternative medicines, and their trials with different herbs and nutritional supplements, some of which have no medical value whatsoever.

There is, however, something inherently evil about unqualified people speaking of predictable cures for things that may be incurable—and even more so when they promote costly treatments without having submitted their results for scientific evaluation.

I have seen instances where men have talked glowingly on the Internet about the so-called cures claimed by an "expert" in the Philippines who diligently carries out repeated prostatic massages on his long-suffering patients with miraculous effects! This doctor's claims of cures seem incredible to me, yet numerous patients make the long trek to the Philippines especially to consult him, and many offer testimonials as to his "skills."

I do not think that this doctor is necessarily an outright fraud, because I suspect there may be substantial benefits in the frequent, and repeated, prostate massages he advocates. There is something wrong, however, with this whole scenario. Diseases such as chronic nonbacterial prostatitis almost always take many sessions to control but are never really cured—like a smoker's chronic bronchitis, which will almost always reoccur from time to time. Besides, this doctor's urological credentials could be better.

Thankfully, more traditional urological treatments for prostatitis prevail. I believe, however, that those doctors who administer them should become more creative in their approach to this all-too-prevalent ailment.

Why is this internal gland we know as the prostate so sensitive to pain? Why does it seem to attract bacteria so easily? Why does it swell much more frequently than other glands? Doctors who have chosen to specialize in this field might ask themselves such questions so as to better understand the entire scope of prostate disorders.

They might also ask: Why are structures that are attached to the prostate, like the seminal vesicles (one of the organs that produces some of the ejaculate fluid) or the vas deferens (the tube that transports sperm from the testicles to the prostate), almost without sensation or disease when the gland itself is so susceptible to pain and inflammation?

To best illustrate this point, I should mention my technique for performing a vasectomy. Although I freeze the skin of the scrotum, I am able to pluck out the vas just beneath, clamp it, cut it, then cauterize it—all with no extra anesthetic. I have also seen men with large cysts on their seminal vesicles, or impressive distensions of them, who have experienced no pain at all. Like the vas, these vesicles have few nerve endings. The prostate, on the other hand, has many.

When we consider prostate disease, we might look to other organs for help—the lungs, for instance. Indeed, the lungs and the prostate are similar in some ways. Lungs are subject to cancer, degenerative enlargement (emphysema), and infection (pneumonia), just as the prostate can develop cancer, enlargement, or prostatitis. But, lungs are also subject to asthma, bronchiectasis, pleurisy. There may be prostatic equivalents that are, at present, all lumped together under the umbrella we know only as prostatitis.

This should lead urologists to expand their thinking on this topic—that there could be more than merely three conditions that can adversely affect the prostate.

The presence of certain chemicals may help us do this, too. For instance, one of the perplexing facts of human anatomy is that there is more zinc residing in the prostate than any other location in the body. No one seems to know why this is or if the quantity of zinc is a factor in disease development. This may also be true of other trace metals, including cadmium or copper.

We know, too, that the protein made by prostate cells—the all-important PSA—makes the gelatinous ejaculate liquid, but again, we cannot ascertain how important this is to fertility. We have also discovered that the seminal vesicles mysteriously manufacture a fruit-sugar substance called "fructose," and that a sperm taken from the testicle or epididymis before contact with the prostate or seminal vesicle can create a normal baby. But the precise details of these phenomena are still mysteries.

What then is the meaning of these findings within the prostate and the attached seminal vesicles? It is important that we know the answers to these questions so we can find out if, perhaps, there is a disease that is related to zinc disturbances that can affect the prostate, or if a muscle disorder, like asthma, can specifically attack prostate cells. In this case, prostatic duct disorders, like a bronchiectasis, might be more significant than we think.

Other relevant questions are these: Could frequent, almost daily, prostatic massages make a difference to prostate health, and should a more vigorous massage under an anesthetic become a serious consideration for long-term treatment? Can chemical cautery, with alcohol or phenol, destroy nerve endings and relieve symptoms? Can the direct infusion of drugs into the prostate, with ultrasound guidance, play a role in the future treatment of enlargement and prostatitis, even cancer?

With answers to these questions urologists might be able to further refine their craft and determine the entire spectrum of prostate ailments—and, more importantly, treatments.

Finally, prostatitis only needs the exclusive attention of a urologist when it is acute and requires surgical drainage, which must be done in a hospital under the supervision of a urology team. Chronic prostatitis, on the other hand, merely requires an empathetic family physician who is willing and able to carry out simple diagnostic measures, provide pragmatic support, and demonstrate the way to recovery.

On this note, there is no need for despair. Remember that, if ever your condition is diagnosed as severe prostatitis, you should afford your treatment a proper chance to succeed. Don't expect overnight miracles.

11. Prostate cancer: Who will get it and why?

Unless medical science advances, and diets and lifestyles change, 14 percent of all males born each year in the early part of the twenty-first century will develop prostate cancer—the second most common cancer in all males, and one that is outnumbered in terms of cases only by skin cancer. About 20 percent of these same males will actually die from the disease. As a killing cancer, prostate cancer is second only to lung cancer.

In the United States, of just under 200,000 men in whom the disease is newly diagnosed this year, approximately 40,000 will succumb to it. And according to the Canadian Cancer Society, each year more than 16,000 Canadian men will be told they have prostate cancer. It will kill more than 3,000 of them.

All this, of course, is the bad news. The good news is that, thanks to the strides science has been able to make over the past two decades, such a death rate need not occur at all. One of the main problems with prostate cancer is that it often masquerades as either an enlarged prostate or a simple case of prostatitis. When in its infancy, cancer may cause no symptoms at all. Nonetheless, early diagnosis and the correct medical or surgical treatment often translate into a complete cure.

All of this must be considered in another light. Those men who are killed by prostate cancer will be victims of what is known as "the tiger"—a lethal, fast-moving form of the disease—while others will suffer the considerably slower-growing form known as "the pussy cat." Life with a slower-growing prostate cancer is almost always sustained for many years, if not decades, with virtually no ill effects other than the psychological impact.

It is heartening to remember, however, that even those men who have the severest form of this dreaded disease—especially those in their seventies and beyond—usually die *with* it rather than *from* it.

Is prostate cancer an epidemic?

In medicine, we tend to apply the term "epidemic" only to a disease that is widespread and passed from one person to another, like the common cold or an influenza virus. But the word may also be used to define something that is extremely prevalent. Given the numbers, prostate cancer may indeed qualify as an epidemic. A one-in-seven chance of contracting a form of cancer that can be fatal if left untreated is a startling and frightening statistic.

The next point we must consider is this: If prostate cancer *is* an epidemic, how should public health officials—doctors, nurses, administrators, and politicians, to name just a few—deal with it? Urologists, the primary health-care providers for a disease that is so obviously pegged to the growing number of graying baby boomers, could sure use help.

The management of any widely distributed health problem involves five levels of medical activity: health promotion, specific prevention, early diagnosis and treatment, disease limitation, and rehabilitation. Some of these are concurrent, while others are sequential. I discuss each in its turn. Meanwhile, let me talk about the preventative measures I feel comfortable in touting: the ongoing issue of genetic predisposition and the possibility that in the not-too-distant future the disease may finally be licked by genetic manipulation that could entail a simple inoculation.

The chemistry of prostate cancer

The biochemical changes in a man's body that promote the development of prostate cancer are just beginning to be understood. It is a complex topic and one which medical scientists can now explain, though not in its entirety.

The prostate gland develops under the influence of the natural male hormone testosterone, which is manufactured in the testicles and ever-present in the adult male. It is this, after all, that promotes not only sexual appetite, but the capacity to satisfy it, too.

Ironically, with the good comes the bad. Testosterone also increases the propensity for prostate cancer, as we know from the fate of those eunuchs who were castrated before puberty. Those young men developed prostate glands all right, but without the presence of testosterone, they did not develop prostate cancer.

Testosterone in the blood circulation is largely fixed to a protein called sex hormone–binding globulin (SHBG). A small amount, however, floats freely and makes its way into the nucleus of the prostate cells.

Cancer starts with the transformation of a normal glandular cell into a malignant cell. Theoretically, this change can be seen under the microscope within the nucleus of the cell. I say theoretically because the very first change in the very first cell cannot be seen. It would be like finding the needle in the haystack.

Actually, cancer is considered to be multifocal in origin. It is not just one cell but a number of cells that become cancerous, and each cell multiplies repeatedly. By the time a microscope can detect the cancer there are thousands, hundreds of thousands, probably millions of cancerous cells involved. The nucleus of the cancer cell will be larger than its noncancerous counterparts, and there will be a prominent nucleolus, a structure within the nucleus.

There will be variations in cell sizes, particularly a variation in nuclear sizes, with more than the normal numbers of chromosomes. The examination of the numbers of chromosomes within the cell nucleus is called ploidy analysis—diploid signifying a relatively benign nature and aneuploid an aggressive cancer. By the time cancer is detectable as a hard spot within the gland, there will often be several satellite lesions, too.

It is not clear when malignant cells leave the gland and start lesions in other areas of the body. It appears that in some men the disease will occupy almost the entire gland before spreading. In other men, the disease will invade adjacent tissue—the seminal vesicles, bladder neck, or urethra—before spreading beyond the confines of the gland. Some men will have widespread disease, usually in bones, at a time when the disease within the prostate is still minuscule.

With all of these potential variations, rendering proper and accurate advice to patients is not always possible. As a rule, however, a person with a low Gleason Grade cancer (associated with a lower PSA count, with fewer biopsy needles showing cancer with less of the cylinder involved, see pg. 119) has better odds of confined disease than someone in whom these parameters are at the other extreme.

Two cancer-fighting genes also dwell within the gland. One is called p-53, the other retinoblastoma gene. When these genes are damaged, in short supply, or totally absent, as is sometimes the case, cancer is promoted by default—by allowing such cancer-promoting genes as ras proto-oncogene and c-erb B2 to thrive.

Generally speaking, prostate cancer occurs with the activation of one set of genes and the loss of another—the set that had the power to deter a tumor from ever taking root. The cancer spreads with the loss of a cell-adhesion molecule called "E-cadherin" and the release of products that promote new blood vessels. The result of this is that new blood vessels nurture the cancer—and promote its growth.

We are now so certain of this that medical scientists believe that prostate cancer may be controlled by the development of medications that can block the very thing on which tumors may feed, not to mention spread.

Health promotion and prostate cancer

Can good health habits, a healthy diet, exercise, freedom from anxiety and malnutrition, an optimistic outlook, lots of laughter, family support, religious faith, community spirit, clean living, vitamins, herbal preparations, and products from "alternative medicine" lower the risks of developing prostate cancer?

None of these factors have undergone trials, nor can we expect them to. It is generally accepted that trials would be far too time-consuming for the amount of information they would unearth. Testimonials, meanwhile, are far from scientific, offering only anecdotal evidence.

Any trials examining the use of food additives and herbal preparations do not come under the jurisdiction, nor even the scrutiny, of such government agencies as the Food and Drug Administration in the United States or the Health Protection Branch in Canada. This means that a maverick business person can freely extract the juice of a turnip, let's say, and market it as a product that is claimed—fraudulently—to help a man with prostate cancer. The government can do little about such practices.

Similarly, cold therapy (cryo-surgery) and heat therapy (thermo-surgery) are not controlled by governmental agencies, either: Ice and fire, after all, have been around for centuries, just like food and food additives. Thus, the public has to make a judgment call. It must decide whether it is for or against these often useless products and procedures, assessing not only the testimonials of well-meaning citizens, but also what may be thinly disguised promotions by entrepreneurial, sometimes unscrupulous, businesspeople who do not have the public's well-being at heart.

At the same time, scientific claims by professionals are notoriously suspect. A headline that announces a finding often befits a tabloid more than a scientific journal.

Let me elaborate. In January 1999, *The Canadian Medical Association Journal* reported a 59 percent increase in the incidence of testicular cancer between 1964 and 1996. Investigative journalists hounded urologists for a likely explanation. After all, such an increase *did* seem alarming and was certainly newsworthy.

In truth, however, the incidence had changed from a mere 4 in 100,000 males to a little more than 6 in 100,000. This was a 59 percent increase all right, but do 2 additional cases per 100,000 really represent a rise that is either catastrophic or cause for alarm? I think not.

Similarly, a prominent Harvard epidemiologist reported a 60 percent increased risk of prostate cancer following vasectomies. A 60 percent increased risk was actually a 4 percent difference in two populations—those with vasectomies and those without.

Repeated studies at other centers failed to confirm these findings. It was like proving that there were more complications with vasectomies done on Tuesdays than there were with those accomplished on Wednesdays. As Mark Twain so astutely observed many years ago, "There are lies, damn lies, and statistics." Indeed, scientists are just as guilty of muddying the water as are product promoters.

As I have expressed my concerns about health-promoting products, let me now state my own prejudices.

I believe that the threat of contracting a disease like cancer—prostate cancer included—forever lingers in the mind of the adult male; actually getting it is increased by both a genetic predisposition to the disease and a weakened immune system. For now, we cannot control the genetic elements of contracting cancer. A weakened immune system, however, is different. It is very definitely a problem we *can* do something about.

In recent years, two interesting revelations have emerged. First, the immune system is affected by a person's emotional state. Thus a happy and optimistic person will have an immune system working for him—fighting for him—while an unhappy, pessimistic man will not have this protection at all. In this respect, the writer Norman Cousins was right: A joke a day may well keep cancer away.

Second, cancer is more likely to start in a body that is teeming with what are known as "free radicals," a hypothesis first put forward by an American scientist named Dr. Denham Harman. According to high-school chemistry, a free radical occurs when a molecule has an unpaired electron in its outer orbit. In medical terms, a free radical is formed when oxygen carried by the hemoglobin in the red blood cells breaks down sugar in other cells to produce energy. In the process, oxygen acquires an extra electron—an unstable state that can be stabilized by the oxidation of fat, protein, or DNA. The oxidation of fat can cause cholesterol deposits on arteries; the oxidation of DNA can promote cancer.

Free radicals, then, cause random damage to protein, enzymes, large molecules, and DNA—an attractive hypothesis that jibes with common sense and provides us with a course of action. Free radicals are akin to rust on a car body that can be delayed or prevented by rust-proofing. By curtailing oxidation with an extra intake of antioxidants, we can neutralize the damage that the free radicals cause in the human body.

Antioxidants are readily available, perhaps most commonly as vitamin C, vitamin E, and beta-carotene. Other sources made familiar to the public include ceruloplasmin, cysteine, glutathione, superoxide dismutase, transferrin, and D-penicillamine. Selenium has an indirect role. A deficiency of it affects the action of glutathione.

It makes sense, then, to adopt a lifestyle that would make a person happier and more optimistic. Exercises and diet help maintain a slim and trim body and contribute to an improved sense of well-being. They may also contribute to a healthier immune system.

An ample intake of vitamin C and vitamin E, and maybe extra glutathione (available, for example, as a milk whey product called Immunocal) or powerful antioxidants, like Pygnogenol, can't hurt. Supplemental selenium also makes sense as a cancer-fighting agent and is available without a prescription.

Specific prevention

Wouldn't it be wonderful if we could prevent prostate cancer the way we can prevent polio, measles, diphtheria, or whooping cough—with a vaccine? Why can't we? Why can't we make a vaccine from cancer cells, inoculate all men in their forties, and thereby prevent all prostate tumors?

There are two simple explanations. First, cancers are as individually specific as the people they attack. Each one is like a fingerprint, possessing its own characteristics that cannot be emulated or duplicated in another person. If, for instance, we could make one person's immune system react to the foreignness of his cancer, it would not follow that we could transfer this response to a second person's cancer, even if both tumors dwelled in the prostate.

Second, cancer cells, though foreign, do not normally provoke an immune reaction as they grow and spread throughout the body. It is curious to me that cancer generally spreads first to the nearest lymph node. As in the case of a bacterial infection, this should ideally be the first garrison of defense.

To put this another way, I am asking myself why cancer runs wild in the lymph nodes when an ordinary infection is not only contained but eliminated by the node's disease-fighting properties. The lymph nodes do not fight, or ward off, cancer cells as they do bacterial invasions. Indeed, cancer cells appear to thrive within them. Until we learn why this happens, a cure for advanced forms of cancer may be a long way off.

Meanwhile, the spread of all cancers really amounts to a breakdown in the established bodily defense mechanism. Forty years ago, scientists wondered if spread (metastatic) cancer in the lymph node could give rise to other cancers (metastases), or whether the metastases always had their origins in primary tumors. In a simple and elegant experiment, an investigator successfully transplanted cancer cells from lymph nodes in laboratory rats into those of other rats of the same genetic strain, proving that metastatic lesions can be the source of cancer in other sites.

Cancer cells can trigger an immune response by being processed by particular cells in the body. These processing cells, or dendritic cells, reside just under the skin. They have been extracted, grown in sterilized bottles outside the body, exposed to irradiated (killed) prostate cancer cells, and then sent back by a series of injections into a patient suffering from the same cancer. An immune reaction against the cancer has been demonstrated, and the cancer has been curtailed or killed. There is justified hope that this kind of approach, called "experimental immunotherapy," will soon lead to the development of a vaccine, but this has yet to depart the experimental stage.

Genetic predisposition

A genetic predisposition to prostate cancer is present in certain unfortunate families. Prostate cancer in a father makes his son twice as likely to develop it, often at a younger age. Prostate cancer in a father and two paternal uncles increases this risk to five times, as does the presence of prostate cancer in three successive generations—great-grandfather, grandfather, and father.

The presence of cancer in two brothers under the age of fifty-five also raises the risk for the third brother, by five times. Furthermore, a recent report from France suggested that prostate cancer in a father made his daughters more likely to develop breast cancer.

What would be the risk of prostate cancer if a father and a maternal grandfather both had it?

I don't know the answer to that. What I *do* know is that these familial cancers have been related to a gene alteration on a specific chromosome that is autosomal—one that is not a sex chromosome.

Actually, it's even a bit more complicated than that. There are a number of genes, called "oncogenes," that promote cancer. There are also suppressor genes that inhibit cancers. The interaction of these—the promoters and the suppressors—within an environment that can be influenced by diet and lifestyle result in a situation that promotes the onset of cancer or, conversely, the curtailment of it.

Race, diet, and lifestyle

Apart from familial predisposition, race and lifestyle are also contributing factors in the contraction of cancer. Studies show that African-American men are 20 percent more likely to develop prostate cancer than white Americans, and at a younger age, too. Japanese men, on the other hand, are less likely to develop prostate cancer, but, as is the case with enlarged prostate, after they have lived in North America for more than twenty years their risk becomes as high as that of white Americans.

By way of further elaboration, the risk of a Japanese man developing prostate cancer while living in the industrial city of Osaka is 6 per 100,000, whereas the risk for an immigrant to San Francisco is 16 per 100,000. Therefore, factors other than genes are thought to play a role—diet, environment, and lifestyle.

Around the world, countries in which animal-fat consumption is high (Sweden, Denmark, Norway, Switzerland, and Belgium, for example) report higher death rates from prostate cancer than countries that have low animal-fat consumption (Japan, Thailand, Taiwan, and the Philippines).

The possibility of some kind of protection in the low-fat Japanese diet has raised a number of hypotheses. Soy products release chemicals called "isoflavones" that may be protectives. Soy also reduces the level of circulating testosterone and blocks the conversion of testosterone into its more potent form, dihydrotestosterone.

Besides the protection offered by soy products, Japanese men consume more vitamin D (found in fish) and substantially smaller amounts of animal fat (found in red meat). It is not clear at this time how much of the protection comes from consuming soy and high levels of vitamin D, or by avoiding juicy steaks.

Tomatoes are known to release a chemical called "lycopene," which is also a protective. For maximum benefit, however, the tomatoes must be cooked in oil, for it is by this method that the important cancer-fighter is released.

If this appears to be an endorsement for spaghetti and pizza, it is. Recently, lycopene has been constituted in capsule form. Several capsules a day are enough to guarantee an intake that is equivalent to a pound or two of tomatoes. A small number of prostate cancer patients have taken large doses of lycopenes and have actually seen their PSA levels fall. Further, there is even early evidence that such high intakes of lycopenes may inhibit the growth of cancers that are already present.

The lycopene story has yet to be fully told, however. What we can surmise is that, just as Japanese men have benefited from fish, Italian men have shown low levels of prostate cancer—probably due to the amount of tomatoes that seems to find its way into Italian cuisine.

Men born with an enzyme deficiency that prevents their testosterone from being converted into the more powerful dihydrotestosterone do not develop prostate cancer. Since this enzyme (5-alpha-reductase) can be inactivated by the drug Proscar (finasteride), it makes sense to wonder if this might not be a chemical preventative for prostate cancer. A widespread study is under way in the United States to compare the effects of Proscar to that of a placebo—an inactive drug that looks identical to the real drug but has no medicinal value. So far, 18,000 men have been enrolled in the study, and results are due in 2005.

A hint that Proscar might make a difference comes from the observation that men who take it show two metabolites (androstenediol glucuronide and androsterone glucuronide) that are similar to those found in Japanese men.

Until a vaccine to prevent prostate cancer is developed, drugs like Proscar, lifestyle changes, genetic manipulation, and dietary supplements remain the best bets in our fight against further development of this fearsome affliction.

12. Prostate cancer: The diagnosis

Back in the 1970s, the early diagnosis of prostate cancer depended exclusively on the rectal examination. The doctor placed his or her gloved and lubricated index finger into the rectum, as he or she does today, and glided it over the back surface of the prostate through the front wall of the rectum to try to feel if the gland had hardened or had formed any irregularities. In this way, enlargement could be discerned. So could a nodule or an asymmetry that might suggest a cancer.

Medical students have always been taught that the surface of the prostate gland should feel like the fleshy part of the hand, and cancer like a knuckle. Thus, when a doctor felt the equivalent of a frozen pea imbedded on the back surface of a prostate, he or she immediately suspected a tumor and arranged for the hard spot to be biopsied.

This biopsy was done by guiding a needle into the hardened area of the prostate with a finger inserted into the rectum to remove a tiny sliver of tissue that could be sent to the laboratory for pathological examination. Sometimes the urologist performed a biopsy by actually making an incision between the scrotum and the anus, under either a local or a general anesthetic, and retrieving a sample of prostate tissue with a scalpel.

The size of the hardened area suggested whether the cancer was confined to the prostate or had spread beyond its wall. Total removal of the gland—a radical prostatectomy—was inevitably recommended when the disease was confined to the prostate. But it was considered inappropriate if it wasn't. In this case, other forms of nonsurgical treatment were immediately set in motion.

One might wonder about the value of the digital rectal examination as it is obvious that only the posterior aspect of the gland can be palpated by the examining finger. The fact is, however, that 70 percent of all prostate tumors originate in this area.

Both the diagnostics of prostate cancer and the treatment of tumors confined to the gland became medical issues in the early 1980s, when Dr. Willet Whitmore—one of North America's most highly respected urological cancer surgeons, and chief of urology at Memorial Sloan-Kettering Hospital in New York City—reviewed and reported his results of radical prostatectomies. Then considered the definitive treatment for a tumor, Dr. Whitmore claimed that his successes by this surgery were infrequent. Many patients he thought he had cured with radical prostatectomies developed recurrent cancer some years later.

This led Dr. Whitmore to question the value of removing a man's prostate. He wondered if those patients who had been cured by this surgery might have done just as well without it. He also considered the possibility that those patients who had died of prostate cancer following a prostatectomy might not have been helped by it, either.

His famous statement, which rings like a Zen koan—"If it's curable, is it necessary? And when necessary, is it curable?"—became known as Whitmore's Conundrum. Following the release of his report, many perfectly reputable urologists around the world gave up radical prostatectomies and referred those patients with localized cancer to their radiotherapy colleagues.

Meanwhile, it was obvious that more accurate diagnostic tools than the index finger were needed to ascertain the extent of a tumor. As a result, that simple blood test we know as the PSA was developed. It would subsequently change the face of urological diagnostics.

A Buffalo, New York, clinic-cum-research center called Roswell Park gets much of the credit for this test, but as in the case of most scientific innovations, honors should have been distributed more widely—on a global basis, in fact. The Japanese scientist Dr. M. Hara first defined a protein that could liquify the gelatinous semen. Dr. L. M. K. Chung and his colleagues were the first to show that this protein was specific to the prostate gland, and it was they who named it "prostate specific antigen." Back in Buffalo, meanwhile, Dr. M. C. Wang and his associates had established the usefulness of this blood test.

Shortly afterward, and back in Japan, Dr. Watanabe was working diligently in his Kyoto clinic to make transrectal ultrasound examinations of the prostate gland meaningful. At Johns Hopkins, Dr. Patrick Walsh was busy clarifying the nerve bundle that he thought was responsible for retaining erection. He developed an anatomical approach to the radical prostatectomy, which was the beginning of what we now call the "nerve-sparing" operation—a procedure that enables some potent men to retain their erectile capabilities after surgery and almost all others to control their urine so they do not suffer the indignity of incontinence.

Today, most knowledgeable patients are as familiar with their PSA results as they are their cholesterol levels, blood pressure readings, and weight fluctuations. So much so that they have been heard to exchange them—like hockey scores or golf handicaps—in clinics across the world.

Interpreting the PSA level

As we discussed earlier, PSA is a protein secreted by every prostate gland cell and is responsible for making the gelatinous ejaculate liquid. If it were a protein secreted exclusively by prostate cancer cells it would be the perfect indicator, or marker. Even as it is, it's a reasonable marker because cancer cells secrete PSA into the bloodstream ten times more than do normal prostate cells.

A PSA reading is a machine-generated analysis of a small amount of blood taken from the patient's forearm, where the veins are most accessible. A level of 4 nanograms per 1 milliliter seems to have become the "magic" figure. Readings below this are, for most men, associated with prostate glands that do not harbor a cancer. Those at or above it are suspect.

Unfortunately, 20 percent of prostate cancers are not associated with an increased release of PSA at all, and this complicates the issue. Furthermore, PSA readings will be higher when:
- there are more prostate cells, as in an enlarged prostate;
- the cells are irritated, as in prostatitis;
- there is a sudden loss of blood flow to a part of the prostate, causing the equivalent of a "heart attack" of the gland, a condition known as prostatic infarct.

Guidelines that have evolved during the last decade relate the level of a man's PSA count to his age, the size of his prostate, and how *rapidly* this count has increased over time.

In a system known as "age-adjusted" PSA, a man under fifty ideally has a reading of less than 2.5. If he is under sixty, it should be less than 3.5, under seventy less than 4.5, and under eighty less than 6.5. In other words, men in these age brackets with "ideal" PSA readings may have low-level cancers that need not be treated. Conversely, they may not have cancer at all.

Unfortunately, some of these men may also be among the 20 percent whose prostate tumors are *not* reflected in the level of PSA their prostates secrete, and they may have cancers even though the PSA count indicates otherwise. By way of example, Norman Schwartzkopf's PSA was only 1.2.

This brings us to another kind of reading—one that is related to the density of PSA as it relates to prostate size. The dimensions of the gland are calculated by an ultrasound measurement of width, length, height, and volume (by a simple mathematical formula). When the volume is multiplied by 0.15, it denotes an acceptable PSA reading that is related directly to prostate size.

Finally, a PSA reading causes some concern if it rises by more than 0.75 units per year. Annual increases in the PSA level constitute what is called PSA velocity and, in my estimation, have proven more predictive of cancer than a PSA reading based only on age or gland size.

More recently, a further refinement in the interpretation of PSA readings has evolved. This development is based on the fact that a PSA level that is not protein-bound rises with enlarged prostates, while PSA readings that are actually *bound* to protein are elevated when cancer is present—a more accurate marker. This means that while a man may indeed have a relatively high level of PSA in his blood count, and one that is free and not protein-bound, his problem may be an enlarged prostate rather than a tumor.

A fairly reliable guideline is this: A free to total PSA reading of less than 0.1 usually means cancer. If the ratio is more than 0.25, it is likely that the patient is cancer-free but has an enlarged prostate.

There is heated debate within the medical community as to whether every man beyond middle age should undergo regular PSA testing. Both the American Cancer Society and the American Urological Association say he should. They favor annual testing for all men starting at age fifty, and at age forty for those who have a family history of prostate cancer. These established medical bodies also agree that *all* African-Americans need to begin monitoring at around forty.

Those opposed to universal testing contend that this kind of screening will prove too expensive, will not necessarily translate into longer lives, and will create a population of disillusioned men who are upset that PSA screening led them to medical procedures that left them with problematic side effects, like bed-wetting and erectile dysfunction.

Where do I stand on this question? There is no doubt in my mind that PSA testing has permitted the earlier diagnosis of prostate cancer. In fact, it has been known to pick up early cancers twice as often as digital rectal examinations. I admit, however, that such widespread PSA testing has led to many more prostate gland removals than necessary. All too often men have suffered some of the nasty side effects the opponents to universal screening are concerned about—varying degrees of incontinence and erectile dysfunction on the one hand, and complications with their incisions on the other.

Those same opponents also claim that indiscriminate PSA testing has sent some men into ill-advised and drastic surgery that ended their lives. On this point I must set the record straight. The number of deaths from prostate surgery of any kind—including radical prostatectomies—has declined so drastically over the years that they are now almost unheard of. Furthermore, in the same period, the death rate from prostate cancer itself has also dropped dramatically, and this has been due directly to the very thing those opponents have opposed—widespread PSA tests as an early diagnostic method.

While some dissenters claim that the drop in prostate cancer deaths is directly related to lower levels of animal fats found in our foods, I must take issue once again. The death rate has fallen most dramatically in those parts of the United States and Canada where radical prostatectomies are carried out as a matter of routine for younger men with proven prostate cancer. Indeed, I honestly believe that early diagnosis translates into higher rates of cure, and that PSA screening contributes to this success. So I must reinforce my point—every man should have an annual PSA test and an annual digital rectal examination from the age of forty or fifty, depending on his family history and ethnic background.

Annual rectal examinations and PSA tests for all men between fifty and seventy (and even younger for those with a family history of prostate cancer) were once supported by the Canadian Urological Association. Then, the organization's executive changed its mind, deciding that there was no hard evidence that such universal testing could be justified, and recommending PSA testing only for men with prostate-related symptoms, or for those who asked.

There is a covert suggestion in the association's recommendation that if a man has no symptoms he is unlikely to have prostate cancer. As we now know, however, this is far from the truth. My colleagues and I have seen numerous patients who delayed PSA testing because they had no symptoms and were shocked to find their levels severely elevated when they finally had the test done. On biopsy, many of these men had advanced cancer and angrily asked why the PSA testing had been discouraged. I had no good answer for them.

The second aspect of the recommendation that suggests testing only for "those men concerned about prostate cancer" begs two questions: "Who isn't concerned about prostate cancer?" and "Who shouldn't be concerned about it?"

Is this policy an attempt by the association to restrict PSA testing to the more-aware elite? I think the association should rethink its stance and I have told it so.

Once and for all: Even though prostate cancer is generally slow-growing, statistics show that the early detection of prostate cancer through early and regular PSA testing has saved and improved many lives.

Ultrasound imaging

When a patient's PSA reading is out of the normal range and/or the rectal examination has revealed a prostatic abnormality that suggests a tumor, ultrasound imaging comes into play. It is widely used to ascertain if a biopsy is warranted.

Fishermen use ultrasound to detect the presence of fish. Gynecologists use it to discern the sex of an unborn child. Kidney stones can be located with ultrasound and assessed in terms of their size and the degree of blockage they are causing within the urinary tract. Suspicious lumps on such organs as the liver and the kidneys can be categorized by ultrasound and diagnosed as being either cancerous tumors or more innocent fluid-filled cysts. Damaged blood vessels, like aneurysms, can also be assessed by ultrasound, allowing specialists to decide on ways to replace or repair them.

Ultrasound imaging of the prostate gland with a rectal probe has come a long way since Dr. Watanabe got his patients to sit on an erect probe in his Kyoto clinic twenty-five years ago. His first efforts showed no more than a few bumps on the surface of the prostate that suggested asymmetry. But it was a start, and one that showed how sound waves could be used in urology to wonderful advantage.

As I've mentioned, the human ear hears sound waves of between 20 and 20,000 vibrations per second, while dogs can hear vibrations well over 20,000 cycles per second. Today's ultrasound equipment can bounce an incredibly high number of sound waves—7.5 million vibrations a second, in fact—well beyond any animal's capacity to hear.

More important is that the ultrasound can "see" well inside a gland as the waves bounce off fat, glandular tissue, muscle, and cancerous tissue in different ways. The results of an ultrasound examination can be made to form images on a television screen that are invaluable to specialists like radiologists, obstetricians, and urologists.

The degree of echogenicity—that is, the "bounce" of the ultrasound waves off different types of tissue—has a characteristic pattern. Thus the image obtained on the screen clearly depicts the contour of the prostate gland because the bounce off surrounding fat is quite different from the bounce off solid tissue. Adjacent structures like the seminal vesicles, urethra, and bladder are also clearly delineated.

The prostate gland itself is projected onto the screen as a mottled gray organ, with the inner part easily distinguishable from the outer part. Within the outer part there may be areas that look darker (hypoechoeic) or lighter (hyperechoeic).

Tumors most often show up on an ultrasound screen as dark spots, or hypoechoeic areas. Some cancers, however, are gray and some light. Whatever their textures, they are usually quite discernible to the urologist and are invaluable in helping to decide the next step in the management of suspected prostate cancer.

13. Prostate cancer: The biopsy, and when it is positive

With the help of modern technology, not only are urologists able to capture images of organs on their screens, they can also use this image to ensure more accurate biopsies than those done twenty years ago.

Ultrasound is absolutely invaluable when the need for a definitive biopsy arises—not to show pictures or shapes of the prostate, but to help a specialist penetrate the tumor with a biopsy needle. Sound waves can show a target at which a biopsy needle must be aimed. From experience, it's a bull's-eye every time because ultrasound also guides the way.

When biopsies are performed, the needles are directed not only at the suspicious areas, but into other regions, too. This is to ensure that the entire gland is being carefully scrutinized for cancer.

Needle one goes into the apex of the left side of the prostate, needle three into the outer mid-body on the gland's left side, and needle five into the left base close to the bladder. Needles two, four, and six go into corresponding areas on the right side of the prostate.

These six biopsies are made by lining up the dots seen on the screen, which indicate where the needle will traverse, and firing the spring-loaded gun into the dots' path. The needle is shot in with such speed that there is no stretching of tissue, which is the main cause of pain. Needles driven in slowly, as was the case with that finger-directed biopsy, stretch tissue and make for a very painful procedure.

What we now call transrectal ultrasound-guided needle biopsies thus allow precise, multiple, and less painful biopsies than those performed twenty years ago.

Patients are prepared for this procedure with a course of antibiotics that starts the evening before the test and usually continues for about two days after it. Lower bowel clean-out with an enema used to be routine just before the biopsy, but this has since been abandoned as unnecessary.

For the actual procedure, the patient is told to lie on his side, curled up in the fetal position, with his knees as close as possible to his chest. A finger examination of his prostate is done first, and this will lubricate and dilate the passage in preparation for the probe, which is wider than any finger. Measurements of the prostate are taken at this time, and a thorough ultrasound examination follows. This will take no more than a few minutes.

The needle-loaded gun for the biopsy is placed in the shaft that runs through the probe, and the patient is instructed not to move. The gun is fired when the directing dot lines up—indicating where the biopsy needle must traverse in order to get a meaningful sample. The needle is then withdrawn, but the probe is left in place. The needle is reinserted for the other five biopsies.

Bleeding from the needle sites is usually minimal, but on rare occasions it can be quite significant. I have not been impressed with any quick measures to lessen this, such as applying finger pressure to the prostate through the rectum. In any case, bleeding following a biopsy is always temporary. Those patients who have been on such blood-thinners as Aspirin and anticoagulation drugs, however, are told to stop taking them about a week before undergoing a prostatic biopsy.

When the gland is particularly large, some prostate centers recommend *more* than six biopsy needles. This makes sense, though in my experience six is quite enough. Most patients are relieved when the gun is fired for the last time and they would be most reluctant to agree to more sessions. When the procedure must be repeated—because of a further and unacceptable rise in the PSA level, for example—patients agree to the test somewhat hesitantly.

When patients are reluctant to subject themselves to repeated biopsies, I do something I think might help them. One of my younger patients, a schoolteacher, bears witness to this. He was fifty-six when he first had an ultrasound-guided biopsy. His PSA score was 5.2, which was high for a man of his age, but the biopsy itself was negative. One year later, however, his PSA was 7.6, and he underwent another biopsy. This was also negative for cancer.

On his own volition, and against my advice, he skipped a year and returned to see me when his PSA score had reached 9.2. A third biopsy was also negative, but a year after this his PSA had soared to 10.7. Another ultrasound and biopsy were recommended, but the patient declined. He'd had enough of the needles, he said, and was willing to take his chances with fate.

I understood this perfectly and felt we might try something a little more comfortable. Even though he'd had no problems with his urine flow I persuaded the man to take Proscar (finasteride), and it worked. Six months later his PSA was 6.3—40 percent lower!

We agreed the patient should have another PSA in six months, and, if the level had dropped by another 10 percent, I could consider it unlikely that we were dealing with cancer. I have made this recommendation in similar circumstances a few times since, and those patients unfortunate enough to require repeated ultrasound-guided biopsies are extremely grateful for it.

Now, I have an understanding with these men. We will agree to further biopsies only if, after having taken Proscar, the PSA has not dropped by predetermined amounts—by 40 percent after six months, or by 50 percent after one year.

The biopsy result

I would be remiss if I did not elaborate here on the role of the pathologist. In urology, as in most other medical disciplines, he or she is indispensable.

A pathologist is a medical doctor who has spent a minimum of five years in specialized training after medical school and has qualified as an expert by passing stringent examinations. The pathologist is often asked, by all manner of hospital doctors, to examine tissue samples and render an opinion on what may be wrong with them. By touch, by sight, or by closer scrutiny under a microscope, he or she can make a valuable pronouncement on the presence or absence of all kinds of diseases, the nature of them, and their seriousness.

When it comes to urology, pathology is a vital link in the chain of treatments that the medical team may have prescribed to any one of their patients. Pathologists do a particularly admirable job for us because they are the final arbiters in defining prostate cancer. When a pathologist is asked to rule prostate cancer either in or out, he is, in effect, basing an opinion entirely on those six slivers of tissue the urologist has sent him—pieces of flesh that resemble six lengths of thread, each about half an inch (1 cm) long.

Almost without exception, the pathologist's biopsy results are returned from the laboratory within a week or two, although it is possible to have the tissue processed within hours or days. The pathologist's report will indicate one of three findings:

- negative—no cancer
- the presence of what we call prostatic intraepithelial neoplasia (PIN)—which means that the biopsy has detected some tissue changes that indicate cancer may be developing
- positive—the absolute presence of cancer

There are, however, some other elements to consider. Negative biopsies may show changes associated with an enlarged prostate, or even prostatitis. In the ultrasound, prostatitis is never clearly indicated but is more definitely proven in the biopsy, when inflammatory cells are seen by the pathologist to have invaded the prostate.

You may ask why the biopsy isn't automatically done to detect prostatitis. The answer is really quite simple: It would too often be hit or miss. That is, the urologist wouldn't know where to steer his needle in his search for prostatitis because the ultrasound wouldn't provide him with a path. So, when prostatitis is found during a biopsy, the needle has made a serendipitous discovery, useful though it is.

It is more important to remember here that while low-grade PIN has almost no significance, high-grade PIN is often premalignant.

The distinction between low- and high-grade PIN, by the way, is a tricky problem for pathologists. I have had slides designated high-grade by one pathologist and low-grade by another. When this controversy occurs in the midst of a rising PSA it can provoke enormous anxiety for the patient, and it is left to me to reiterate the bottom line as I have come to know it—that 50 percent of all patients with high-grade PINs eventually develop prostate cancer.

One of my patients, a colleague physician, is walking testimony to the confusion—not to mention the anguish—that a high-grade PIN can provoke. He was forty-six when he first came to see me, after having run a routine PSA blood test on himself, of all things. He was alarmed when the biochemistry laboratory told him it was 6.4. He was *certain* he had cancer.

My ultrasound-guided biopsy on him, however, revealed only a high-grade PIN, but another PSA blood test, done at the hospital six months later, indicated a reading of 7.2! His PSA was rising.

A repeat biopsy was arranged, and again the results for cancer were negative, though two of the six biopsy specimens still showed a high-grade PIN. At this point, I had the slides reviewed by Dr. Jonathan Epstein at Johns Hopkins, a recognized authority on PIN. He felt that a high-grade PIN had been too strong a diagnosis and that the patient's grade really bordered on being low.

The patient, meanwhile, was so preoccupied with the possibility of cancer that he was no longer able to work. He thought this was inevitable so he asked me to remove his prostate. There was no indication that such drastic surgery was needed, I said. However, I informed him that I might accede to his wishes if he gave me explicit consent. He did. Later, when I reviewed his chart, I suspected that he would almost certainly have developed cancer and was probably better off having the surgery now than when he was older—particularly since his state of mind had been so adversely distorted by his obsession that he was in danger of losing his wife and his career.

Two years after first seeing this man, I performed the operation. The pathology report on the removed prostate revealed the presence of a high-grade PIN, but there were still no signs of cancer. Nonetheless, the patient never regretted the operation and, fortunately, suffered no major side effects.

The PIN report

Assessing PIN is a relatively new way pathologists have agreed to define cell changes in the biopsy specimens received from urologists. The technique entails examining slices of the specimens they have obtained under a microscope. Once they are convinced that cancer is absent, they look for nuclear changes that occur when cells multiply more quickly than they should—like variations in nucleus size and the presence of highly staining structures called nucleoli. PIN is read as low-grade, which is innocuous, or high-grade, which is considered pre-malignant.

More important for you to remember is that, if repeat biopsies show PIN only, careful follow-up is still necessary, with regular or semi-annual PSA tests—even more so if the PSA climbs more than 0.75 units in one year. Half of those patients who undergo repeated biopsies because of a high-grade PIN show some degree of cancer.

The Gleason Grade

While the biopsy indicates the presence of cancer, other information is required to determine its type, character, and severity. This brings us to the Gleason Grade, so called because it was devised by an American pathologist named Dr. Donald Gleason more than twenty years ago. Since then it has become the international standard by which prostate cancer is measured and described.

To put this another way, prostate cancer is reported in terms of the Gleason Grade, which is a score between 2 and 10. The pathologist may also report the percentage of cancer involved within the tiny cylinder of tissue he has been sent to examine.

So, the Gleason Grade is really a pathologist's opinion of the degree of differentiation in cancer cells, and it is one that influences the urologist's plan of action.

Coupled with the PSA, the Gleason Grade gives a urologist the most valuable information he or she requires to be able to arrive at a prognosis. Once the seriousness of cancer and the extent to which it may have spread are known—the stage of the disease—the proper way to manage it can be assigned.

The degree of cell-differentiation is the key to how well a patient is likely to fare with the disease. Usually, one who has a well-differentiated tumor will do better than one who has a poorly differentiated tumor.

Obviously, there is no point in removing a patient's prostate gland without removing all of his cancer, so it's important to determine if surgery is the answer to his problems or whether he might be better served by other treatment. Before we can do this, we must study the Gleason Grade carefully. Its goal, after all, is to help ascertain which cancer will need immediate treatment and which kind won't need immediate treatment at all.

How the pathologist assigns the Gleason Grade

The pathologist determines the presence of prostate cancer when he sees changes in the appearance of certain cells. Compared to ordinary, healthy cells, cancer cells have a more variegated nucleus—they are not uniform in their sizes, shapes, and clusters. They also show prominent disfiguration within the nucleus itself. Pathologists determine this information by seeing how clusters of cells stain differently from normal cells.

Perhaps I may make the Gleason Grade more comprehensible by suggesting an analogy between the pathological grading and the box of raspberries. If you can imagine prostate tissue under the microscope looking rather like a box of freshly picked raspberries lying among leaves and twigs, you might be able to understand what a thin cross section of such a box might look like. Different raspberries would be cut in different places so that more or less of their central cavities will be seen. Some will be cut at their tips, others at their bases, some in cross sections, others obliquely.

The term the pathologist uses to describe the raspberries is *acini*, cell clusters so shaped that they each have a central cavity. The twigs and leaves, meanwhile, are the supporting tissue, which the pathologist calls *stroma*.

- Gleason Grade 1 cancer is when there are more berries—or cell clusters—relative to the amount of twigs, or stroma, in the box. This is what pathologists call "a decreased amount of stroma." In this case, there are no berries—or cell clusters—stuck together, nor do the berries, or cell clusters, vary in size.

- Gleason Grade 2 cancer is when the raspberries—or cell clusters—are of different sizes. This is not to be confused with berries cut high or low and thus giving an appearance of different sizes. A slice of a box of raspberries of different sizes should be distinguishable from one with uniform size. In pathological terms, this would be described as "variation in glandular size or variation in size of acini."

- Gleason Grade 3 cancer describes a situation where three or four raspberries—or cell clusters—have come together and are not just lying adjacent to one another but are actually stuck together. The berries, or cell clusters, are so well bonded that the hairs on them at the point of contact are undetectable.

- Gleason Grade 4 cancer is when five or more berries coalesce, and the descriptive term pathologists use for this is "cribriform pattern of invasive cancer." In our box of raspberries, this would signify the further loss of hair.

The Gleason Grade

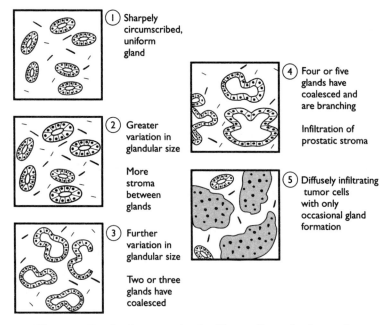

1. Sharply circumscribed, uniform gland

2. Greater variation in glandular size

   More stroma between glands

3. Further variation in glandular size

   Two or three glands have coalesced

4. Four or five glands have coalesced and are branching

   Infiltration of prostatic stroma

5. Diffusely infiltrating tumor cells with only occasional gland formation

- Gleason Grade 5 cancer looks like a slice of a box of raspberries that has been stepped upon. Any evidence of the hollow part of the berry is lost. Almost all of the fruit has been completely crushed.

In assigning the Gleason Grade, the pathologist takes the two most predominant patterns seen under his microscope and adds them together. If, for example, he sees no more than two to three raspberries joined together, he safely determines this to mean grade 3. If he sees no other pattern—such as more berries joining—he calls it 3 and 3, assigning a grade of Gleason 6 … and so on down the line.

The pathologist uses a few tricks to clarify confusing scenarios. If, for instance, he is not sure if he is looking at a prostate cell, he can stain for PSA. If the cell picks up the PSA, it has to be a prostate cell. Also, when he is not certain if the acini are merely touching, or coalescing, he can stain for the equivalent of the hairs on the berries. This is the cytokeratin stain and, when absent, suggests the presence of cancer with all its invasive features.

From this description it should be apparent that the most subtle difference lies in distinguishing Gleason Grade 3 from Gleason Grade 4, and this is the distinction that may be the most significant.

Cancer patients often ask me, somewhat hopefully, if the pathologist could have been mistaken in his opinion. Could he have diagnosed a cancerous tumor when there wasn't one? This, I explain, is indeed possible. Pathologists are human, after all. But it does not happen often—in fact, it rarely happens at all.

It is also possible for the slides of one person to be mistaken for the slides of another, but there are a number of safeguards to protect against such accidents, and for the most part they work well.

From the urologist's standpoint, Gleason Grades of 6 and lower are considered to denote low-grade tumors or those that are slow-growing—the "pussy cats." Grades 8, 9, and 10 are considered to depict high-grade aggressive tumors—the "tigers." Gleason Grade 7, meanwhile, is categorized separately as an entity unto itself because it could probably have been either a 6 or an 8. Usually, I exercise caution by calling a Gleason Grade 7 a Gleason Grade 8 and prescribing treatment accordingly.

Staging

When prostate cancer has been diagnosed in a patient, with a pathological level of differentiation that has been reflected by the Gleason Grade, the next stage is a series of evaluations aimed at determining the extent of his cancer. This is a process called staging, and it is done in one of two ways:

- the ABC method, which dates back to 1960s
- the TNM method, which was introduced in 1992

Because the TNM method is the more widely accepted form today, I will describe it here with the ABC equivalent in parentheses.

- T1a (A1) means that the tumor was found by chance in the prostate and that it occupies less than 5 percent of the tissue excised during surgery.
- T1b (A2) means that more than 5 percent of the excised tissue is cancerous.
- T1c (A3?) means that cancer was found on a needle biopsy done because the PSA was elevated, not because it was suspected on rectal examination.
- T2a (B1) means that a tumor was suspected on digital rectal examination, but that it is confined to less than one-half of one lobe.
- T2b (B2) means that cancer was suspected on digital rectal examination and involves more than half of one lobe.
- T2c (B3) means that the cancer has spread to both lobes.
- T3a (C1) means the cancer has spread outside the capsule on one side.
- T3b (C2) means that the cancer has spread beyond the capsule on both sides.
- T3c means the cancer has spread to one or both seminal vesicles.
- T4 means the cancer has spread to adjacent tissue like the bladder neck or urethra.

In advanced staging, when the cancer has spread beyond the prostate—first into the lymph nodes, and later into bones and other organs—we use other designations:

- N0 means there is no lymph node involvement.
- Nx means the nodes cannot or have not been evaluated.
- N1 means that cancer is present, but that the involved

node—or nodes—has enlarged by less than three-quarters of an inch (2 cm).

- N2 means that cancer has enlarged one, or more, nodes by more than three-quarters of an inch (2 cm).
  (The ABC method calls all these categories D1.)
- M means that there is widespread cancer, probably now in the bones.
- M0 means no distant metastases.
- Mx means distant metastases have not, and cannot, be evaluated.
- M1 means distant metastases.
- M1a means cancer has spread into nodes other than the regional nodes.
- M1b means that the cancer has spread to the bones.
- M1c means cancer has reached sites other than the skeleton, such as the liver.
  (In the ABC equivalent, each of these categories is designated as D2.)

Bone scans and others

When we are fairly certain that the cancer has spread beyond the prostate, we must find out where it has gone and how far it has spread. Ninety percent of the time, cancer that spreads from the prostate into the lymph nodes enters the bone, so the bone scan is absolutely imperative in helping us further define the extent of the disease.

(It would be wonderful if urologists had a test that showed whether or not cancer had invaded the lymph nodes themselves, but short of surgical explorations there are, as yet, no other accurate methods.)

A bone scan used to be routine before treatment in every

prostate patient. Recently, though, it has been suggested that when the Gleason Grade is under 6, and the PSA reading is under 10, it is unnecessary. I agree.

The bone scan for cancer begins with an intravenous injection of a radioactive material that goes directly to the skeleton. Three hours later the patient is scanned from head to toe, a procedure that takes about one hour. The radioactive material emits gamma rays that produce the equivalent of an X-ray picture of the bones. When cancer is present, the affected areas show up as dark spots.

Some centers insist upon a CT scan for every prostate cancer patient, as well as a bone scan. The CT scan can detect when lymph nodes have been enlarged by more than half an inch (1 cm) in either length or width, which immediately raises the suspicions of cancer. The problem is that nodes that are smaller than this can be cancerous, too. So a CT scan does not always help in defining the extent of the disease.

Cancerous changes within the prostate gland itself cannot be detected either by a CT scan or by a nuclear magnetic scan. Consequently, I don't consider the CT scan helpful in staging this disease at all, but most radiotherapists consider it mandatory before treatment is begun.

Finally, it should now be apparent that once prostate cancer has been diagnosed, it is not a simple case of "on with the surgery." Far from it. What kind of treatment is best for which patient will ultimately depend on age, general health, attitude, or a combination of all three—and the type and extent of the cancer we are trying to contain.

14. Prostate cancer: Managing the disease

As I have demonstrated, no urologist wants to subject a prostate cancer patient to a radical prostatectomy unless it is going to achieve the desired result. Sometimes, though, there is no choice. A relatively young, healthy man with the "tiger" must obviously have aggressive treatment. So must a young man with the "pussy cat"—to ensure that his cancer will not become less manageable later.

For older men who might not be able to withstand such major surgery, alternative treatment plans must be mapped out. These are usually done with one important factor in mind: Because prostate cancer is nearly always slow-growing, many of these patients will live out the rest of their lives with it and without too many ill effects.

In other words, why let surgery affect the well-being of a perfectly active seventy-five-year-old man when his condition can be contained, and to some extent improved, with what we call "palliative treatment." Indeed, most such patients will eventually die from other causes.

Generally speaking, there are five ways to treat prostate cancer, but the decision as to when to apply these methods can be complex. Some treatments are considered curative on their own, while others are merely palliative. Also, one treatment may be more successful when it has followed another, or when combined with another. Other procedures, however, are futile when applied sequentially.

Prostate cancer treatments are:

- radical prostatectomy
- nothing at all (watchful waiting)
- hormone treatment
- radiotherapy and brachytherapy
- combination therapy

Radical prostatectomy is the topic of a later chapter.

When I say nothing at all, I must add that I do not mean precisely that. This term applies to another phrase that is often used in medicine—"watchful waiting."

Watchful waiting

During this period of observation—intense or otherwise, depending on age or the severity of the problem—the patient is monitored frequently to make sure that his urinary tract continues to function and to check for signs that his cancer has not become life-threatening.

Does this period of watchful waiting, or no treatment, make any sense?

Swedish experts thought it did. They felt that if prostate cancer was slow-growing, as it so often is, and if many men were dying with it rather than from it, why not simply follow men in whom the disease had been diagnosed and offer treatment only if and when they began to suffer, from pain, perhaps, or from voiding difficulties?

Around the world, this no-treatment option became the accepted one when patients were elderly, usually beyond the age of seventy-five, or for men with fewer than ten years of further life expectancy. With watchful waiting, however, it became apparent that those men with high Gleason Grade cancers did poorly. Their disease advanced quickly, necessitating hormone treatment.

Might they have been better off with earlier treatment, perhaps upon diagnosis? There was no clear-cut message in the medical literature on this point. In fact, the idea was to withhold treatment as long as the patient was symptom-free—delay the deployment of the guns, so to speak, until it became necessary to use them. Why waste the ammunition? It may run out by the time it is really needed. This approach was based on speculation, not science.

To prove this point, a team of British doctors carried out a study on older men who had advanced but symptom-free prostate cancer. Half were treated upon diagnosis, and the other half only when they developed pain. The group that was offered early treatment fared far better. They did not suffer collapsed spines caused by the invasion of cancer. Their urinary tracts remained unobstructed for longer. Their times to further disease, and their times to death, were also delayed. In other words, watchful waiting made very little sense.

Something usually has to be done to help men such as these as soon as prostate cancer is diagnosed. I know this from my experience with a seventy-year-old man who was referred to me with a PSA reading of 8.4, but who had no difficulty urinating. Upon a rectal examination, I suspected cancer on the left side of his prostate, and ultrasound-guided biopsies later revealed Gleason Grades 7 and 8 prostate cancer in three of six needles. The bone scan, however, was negative.

I strongly advised hormone treatment followed by radio-therapy—combination treatment—but the patient elected watchful waiting. Perhaps his decision was influenced by his ethnic origin. (He was Swedish.) There was no way I could get him to change his mind.

One year later, his PSA had risen to 12.8, and it was only then that he agreed to the treatment I had first suggested. Soon, his PSA dropped to 2.0, but a year later it rose to 38.9. A bone scan revealed metastatic lesions in his hips and ribs.

I am sad to report that further hormone treatment failed this man. He managed at home for six years from the time of his diagnosis and was then admitted to hospital for palliative care. He died some weeks later. To my mind, the year he'd spent in watchful waiting cost him his life.

I am much happier to record those occasions when watchful waiting was a more appropriate measure, as evidenced by a sixty-three-year-old businessman on whom I had performed a routine TURP for an enlarged prostate. A Gleason Grade 4 cancer, however, was found in two chips that were sent to the laboratory after his surgery.

When I first disclosed the pathology report to the man, he wanted his prostate removed immediately. "There's no way I can live with the thought of cancer in my body," he said, voicing a common reaction.

I told him his PSA reading (only 2.4) was fairly low and nothing to worry about.

"Why don't we follow the situation with regular PSAs and rectal exams?" I suggested. "There's time enough for surgery should the situation change."

Besides, I added, there was no guarantee that I could preserve his potency, which is something I would have been concerned about if I were in his shoes.

I have followed this patient for more than six years and there has been no detectable progression in his disease, no PSA elevations, no deterioration in his well-being. He is a happy man.

Patients who elect simply to have their situations followed, rather than be treated from the outset, provide us with figures that document their risk of developing more serious complications:

- A man with a Gleason Grade 2, 3, or 4 tumor has a 2 percent chance of having his cancer spread each year.
- When the Gleason Grade is 5, 6, or 7, the chances rise to more than 5 percent annually.
- A Gleason Grade of between 7 and 10 means that the chances of developing metastases are nearly 14 percent per year.

Dr. Alan W. Partin of the Johns Hopkins Medical Center has constructed a table that predicts the probability of prostate cancer being confined to the gland based on the Gleason Grade and the PSA reading. For example:

- If a man has a Gleason score of 7, a PSA reading of 8, and non-palpable disease on rectal examination (T1c disease), his chances of having a tumor confined to his prostate are 50 percent.
- If the Gleason Grade is the same, and the PSA reading is between 10 and 20, the chances of the disease being confined to the gland drop to 35 percent.
- If, with the same Gleason Grade, the PSA score is above 20, the chances drop to 18 percent. This means that there is an 82 percent chance that surgery alone may not cure his problem.

Dr. Partin's table, known simply as the Partin Table, is a useful guide, but decisions on what treatments should be used, based on his calculations, are less straightforward. Some men will choose surgery even though, according to Dr. Partin, they have only a 20 percent chance of a complete cure, while others with a nearly 80 percent chance of eliminating cancer with surgery will decline it.

Many men like to make choices for themselves, while others leave them to their doctors or to their families. It is never an easy decision.

Of course, if watchful waiting fails and the disease worsens, the urological team must order more conventional treatment—and soon.

Hormone treatment

The objective of hormone treatment is to get the patient's testosterone level down to zero—or close to zero—so that it will not help the prostate tumor to grow. (Remember that prostate cancer is thought to be closely related to virility.) It is used mostly when a patient has cancer that has already spread by the time his diagnosis is made.

Hormone treatment consists of:

- orchiectomy—the surgical removal of the testicles;
- an antifungal pill called Nizoral (ketoconazole);
- injections of drugs called LHRH analogues to block testosterone production in the testicles;
- antiandrogen pills that block testosterone from entering prostate cells and prevent it from being made by the adrenal gland.

Calling hormone treatment "palliative" treatment, as is often the case, is unduly pessimistic. Almost all—perhaps 90 percent—men initially respond to it quite positively. Up to 4 percent are actually cured by it, or show no evidence of further disease while having it, while nearly 50 percent stay controlled, or remain in remission for many years as long as they continue to have the treatment.

One of these men, I recall, was a healthy fifty-two-year-old electronics technician who was surprised to learn that his PSA reading was an astounding 83! That's when he first came to see me. My investigations revealed that he had an advanced tumor. An ultrasound-guided biopsy revealed a Gleason Grade 8 cancer in all six needles, and a bone scan was positive in his lower back, too. In effect, this man had M1b or D2 disease.

Hormone therapy was started immediately, and, within only a month or so, the patient's PSA had dropped to 0.24, which is really akin to zero. More than eight years after consulting me, with panic in his face, he has no detectable disease.

He is one of the lucky ones. While, as I have said, half of the patients who have hormone treatment are definitely helped by it, the other 50 percent do not fare as well. They demonstrate slow, but progressive, disease within two years of starting the treatment and, unfortunately, die. I should be quick to add, however, that these men are most often elderly—much older than our electronics technician.

Alas, hormone treatment is by no means a panacea. We know it can help an advanced cancer, but there is often nothing that can be done to alleviate other unrelated health problems. Such was the case with yet another retired physician who sought me out. He had a Gleason Grade 9 cancer with a PSA reading of 21.7. He typified the kind of patient who would profit from hormone treatment, except that after starting it, progressive kidney failure was diagnosed in this patient.

I carried out an orchiectomy on him when his PSA rose to 36, and he quickly found himself in remission with a PSA of zero. Since then, however, his kidneys have deteriorated. Because he is now seventy-eight, all we can do is monitor him carefully with that "watchful waiting" and keep him comfortable

The main advantage of the orchiectomy is that it can reduce a man's testosterone level to what we call "a castrate level" within a matter of hours, while pills and injections may take days, even weeks.

There are two ways to perform this procedure. One is called the bilateral orchiectomy, which means that the entire testicles are removed; the other is known as a subcapsular orchiectomy. In this, the surgeon takes out only the interiors of the testicles, leaving the outer shells. This method is equally as effective as the bilateral one, and in no way compromises treatment because there are no testosterone-producing cells in the outer shells.

The subcapsular removal of the testicles does, however, have the advantage of maintaining a semblance of normal male anatomy—for psychological reasons, if nothing else. If I had to have an orchiectomy to control prostate cancer, I would insist upon a carefully done subcapsular procedure because this operation is less morbid and has fewer complications.

You may ask another of my patients about this—a sixty-two-year-old father of two preteen children whose advanced prostate cancer had already spread into his bones when he arrived at my office. His biopsy showed a Gleason Grade 9.

I performed a subcapsular orchiectomy on him and installed a testicular prostheses in his scrotum because he said he wanted to have a "normal" body so he would not feel awkward when seen naked. He also opted for antiandrogens. Fourteen years after surgery, his PSA is zero, and he's fine, except for the constant fear that his cancer may return.

After the orchiectomy, the next quickest way to lower the testosterone level is by using the antifungal drug Nizoral (keto-conazole). The 200-milligram tablet must be administered in a dosage of 1,200 milligrams per day. With this, castrate levels of testosterone are achieved within twenty-four hours but are maintained only while taking this drug.

The least expensive way to lower the testosterone to castrate level is with the female hormone pill DES (stilboestrol).

Three milligrams per day is the standard dose to achieve this effect in two weeks, but 1 milligram may suffice. This treatment has fallen into disfavor, however, because of cardiovascular complications. DES causes fluid retention and increases the risk of heart attacks and inflamed blood clots in the legs (thrombophlebitis), which may lead to a potentially fatal blood clot in the lungs (pulmonary embolism).

Whenever I prescribe DES, I always tell the patient to take common Aspirin with it to lessen these risks. An anticoagulant like Coumadin (warfarin) may prove equally successful in preventing cardiovascular complications.

Another useful hormone-treatment drug is a progesterone-like hormone pill called Androcur (cyproterone acetate). This has become very popular in Canada and in Europe, although it is not currently available in the United States. It has the dual effect of suppressing testosterone production in the testicles while also blocking its entry into prostate cells. Unlike most hormonal medications, it does not cause hot flashes.

Critics of this particular drug argue that it is less likely to achieve castrate levels of testosterone than other medications or surgery, that a patient's PSA may not fall as low as it might, and that there are increased risks of blood clots, as well as extreme muscle fatigue. Many patients have responded well to it, though, especially when it is taken with small doses of DES (0.1 mg a day). Further, when patients are faced with surgical castration because of their cancer, they nearly always prefer to take a simple pill. When they do well on it, they are generally reluctant to try anything else.

The most popular, yet most expensive, treatment for achieving "medical castration" is the combination of oral antiandrogens and drugs that are injected into the fat beneath the skin or into the muscle. By this method, castrate levels of testosterone are achieved in two or three weeks with only one injection. Thereafter, injections might be given every month, every two months, every three months, or every four months, depending on the particular drug used.

Three pharmaceutical firms compete for this market. Abbott makes Lupron (leuprolide), which comes as a 7.5-milligram monthly intramuscular dose or as a 22.5-milligram intramuscular dose every three months; Hoechst-Roussel makes Suprefact (buserelin), which comes as a 3.3-milligram subcutaneous monthly injection or as a 6.6-milligram subcutaneous injection every two months; Zeneca makes Zoladex (goserelin), which comes as a monthly subcutaneous injection of 3.6 milligrams or as a 10.8-milligram dosage to be injected every three months.

These drugs work by stopping testosterone production in the testicles after first making them overproduce it—in effect stimulating so much of the hormone that further production is exhausted. This initial stimulation of testosterone output—known as the "flare"—might be considered harmful to a patient with prostate cancer since the healthy flow could stimulate the growth of his tumor.

The "flare," meanwhile, can be suppressed by treating the patient with one of several oral antiandrogen preparations for a couple of weeks before administering the first injection. These drugs successfully block testosterone from entering the cancerous prostate cell just as a tarp would prevent water from seeping into a lawn.

The antiandrogens come in two types: steroidal or nonsteroidal. Those that are steroidal, Androcur (cyproterone acetate) and Megace (megestrol acetate), have both a good and a bad side. On the one hand, they prevent hot flashes. On the other hand, they have a cholesterol-like formulation that is associated with phlebitis.

The nonsteroidal antiandrogens, however, are the most popular and the most commonly prescribed. One of these,

Euflex (flutamide), is a pill that must be taken three times a day and is fairly innocuous—causing rare intestinal upsets and even rarer liver damage as side effects. Another medication, Nilutamide (Anandron), is taken three times daily in 100-milligram tablets. Unlike Euflex it has no intestinal side effects at all, although some patients complain that it makes them extra sensitive to sunlight.

Some time ago I was invited by the drug company Hoechst-Roussel to a think-tank session designed to find out why its Anandron was not competing well against Schering's Euflex, and how the company could improve its sales of this very useful drug. It is always difficult, after all, for a company to break into the market with a new drug when an earlier one has become so well established, and when there is no real difference in clinical effectiveness between the two.

The difference here, I'd decided, was solely in each drug's side effects. With this in mind I suggested that Hoechst-Roussel might provide urologists with free sunglasses to give to those patients about to take Anandron. The glasses could serve as a reminder to the urologist to tell the patient that wearing sunglasses—for free, no less!—might be better than suffering cramps and diarrhea, and risking liver damage.

Predictably, the company did not adopt my idea—its management felt it would put too much emphasis on the drug's negative aspects. Later on, without improved sales, those same company officials admitted that I may have had a point.

The third, and most recently available nonsteroidal antiandrogen, is Casdodex (bicalutamide), made by Zeneca. This has the advantage of once-a-day doses—a 50-milligram tablet at a time—and almost no side effects.

The combined use of antiandrogens and injections should maximize the blockage of male hormone effects, and this in turn should improve the prognosis for patients with advanced prostate cancers.

Many studies have been done on the value of using a combination of these pills and injections to block testosterone, but they are divided on the success rates. In a large-scale study done in the United States, both a rising PSA and the time-to-death rate were unaltered by adding antiandrogens to surgical castration. It is still not clear whether the addition of antiandrogen pills to injection treatment prolongs the life of a man suffering from advanced prostate cancer.

More certain is that, while medical castration can be reversed, surgical castration cannot. A stop in the injections will eventually restore the testosterone level, although it may take between three and six months (or even longer) for the hot flashes to disappear or the libido to return.

Investigators in Vancouver, British Columbia, have recently proposed cyclical hormonal therapy, not only for psychological reasons but because the animal experiments they had done suggested that the periodic restoration of a normal testosterone environment kept cancer cells from developing hormone independence.

Put another way: When testosterone is eliminated from the body, certain cancer cells that do not depend on it for survival, and are normally held in check by it, are allowed to flourish. Practically, then, routine hormonal treatment is stopped when a patient's PSA reaches the nadir, or lowest level, so as to allow the testosterone to reappear. The treatment is restarted when the PSA rises again.

This cyclical treatment has yet to be time-tested, but if it is more effective than, or even as good as, continuous treatment, it would represent a strong argument in favor of medical castration over surgical castration. It should also be remembered that by allowing his testosterone to reach a "normal" level, a patient's psychological health is restored.

Historically, there has been no difference in prostate cancer survival rates whether testosterone levels have been lowered by

surgical orchiectomy or controlled by estrogens and progesta-
tional agents or injections. Nor have there been advantages in
adding one modality of treatment to another—giving injections
to a man who has had a surgical orchiectomy, for example, or
estrogens to another who has been getting injections.

What few differences are evident have been seen in the psychological effects on the patient, the medical costs to govern-
ments in those countries where there is socialized medicine,
and a medication's side effects.

Still another way to achieve castrate levels of testosterone is
by using a drug that blocks testosterone production without
first stimulating it. This is the rationale behind Amgen's product—an LHRH antagonist. It has not yet reached the market,
so its effectiveness has yet to be proven. It is attractive, however, because it eliminates the need to take antiandrogen pills
before the injections.

Sometimes, prostate cancer is controlled by hormone treatment, but the plumbing problems aren't. This was the case
with an eighty-two-year-old artist whose biopsy confirmed a
Gleason Grade 8 cancer. His PSA score was 25. Hormone
treatment was started right away, but three months later the
patient could not urinate and I had to perform a TURP on him.

The tissue removed during his surgery showed the same
Gleason Grade score of 8, but his PSA had fallen to zero. It
was still at this level five years later when the man died of
other causes.

Why does advanced prostate cancer in one patient stay under
the control of hormones for years, even decades, while another
patient with a similar cancer succumbs in a matter of months? At
this point nobody knows. It is the subject of intensive research.

When a patient doesn't respond to hormone treatment, further treatment depends upon his overall health. If he is bedridden and in severe pain, analgesics and cortisone preparations,
along with a drug called Mitoxantrone (in doses of 12 to 14

mg per square meter of body surface every three weeks), are all that would be prescribed. Mitoxantrone has been demonstrated to help alleviate pain and, although no reported cures have been ascribed to it, nonetheless contributes to the lengthening of lives.

By the way, for medical purposes a patient's body surface area is calculated on a graph. A line that connects his weight and height intersects a third vertical line that denotes this surface in square meters. This is used a lot in clinical medicine.

Radiotherapy and brachytherapy

Radiotherapy is most effective when it follows a short course of hormone therapy. This combination is called neo-adjuvant therapy, and it is becoming the established treatment when surgery is not the best option.

When it is given first, hormone therapy shrinks the gland and provides a smaller target for radiotherapy later, thus reducing the chances of radioactive spillover into adjacent sites. Furthermore, as recent reports have indicated, the combination of radio and hormone therapy improves results.

Three-dimensional conformal radiotherapy is a term used to describe a computer-assisted configuration of the prostate used to guide the radiation. The prostate gland is more precisely attacked with this technique, and even larger doses of radiation can be administered without overflowing into unwanted areas.

The total cumulative amount of "rads," or centigrays (cGy), is critical. For prostate cancer, about 6,000 cGy must be delivered, usually in about thirty-five treatment sessions, each lasting fifteen minutes. Skipping Saturdays and Sundays, the entire treatment takes about seven weeks. If there is an interruption in the treatment because of an illness, it is not necessary to restart it; the important factor is the total amount of radiation administered over a given period.

Radiation can also be delivered by radioactive pellets, or seeds, that are placed inside the prostate gland itself. This technique is called "brachytherapy." Back in the 1970s, doctors at New York City's Memorial Sloan-Kettering Hospital placed seeds of radioactive iodine into a patient's prostate after exposing the gland with a surgical incision below the navel. The results were not impressive, and the procedure was abandoned.

Brachytherapy resurfaced, however, with the development of ultrasound-guided placement of two kinds of pellets—one containing radioactive iodine, the other radioactive palladium. In this procedure, the patient is placed in an exaggerated child-bearing position. An ultrasound probe is inserted into his rectum and a thick, metal template, with preset holes, is placed on the perineum, the space between the scrotum and anus. The holes in the thick template allow a series of needles to be inserted, parallel and evenly.

The radioactive iodine pellets are placed inside the prostate at varying depths to ensure an even distribution of the radiation they will emit. In one technique, the pellets stay in permanently. In another, the pellets are on a string and are removed when doctors feel that sufficient radiation has been delivered, usually after a few days or weeks.

Palladium seeds are more powerful than radioactive iodine seeds. Consequently, they are used only when the Gleason Grade is 7 or higher.

In another variation of this technique, brachytherapy is combined with radiotherapy that is beamed externally at the draining lymph nodes. To improve results, external radiation doses can be increased at will.

Some patients sail through radiotherapy—beams or seeds—with no side effects whatsoever, while others experience extraordinary fatigue, diarrhea, cramps, and urinary frequency and urgency. These side effects usually start during the second or third week of treatment, peak at five to six weeks, and then subside. Incontinence is hardly ever a consequence, but erectile dysfunction occurs in up to 50 percent of all patients who undergo this treatment, and this can be permanent.

I should also point out that those patients who suffer from erectile dysfunction following radiotherapy do not do so immediately. Rather, the condition is a gradual one that tends to take several years to peak.

What of the other side effects?

In one hospital study, 24 percent of patients who underwent radiotherapy displayed genitourinary symptoms, 43 percent had gastrointestinal symptoms, and about 3 percent had to abandon the treatment because these side effects were severe. Unfortunately, adverse side effects can continue to resurface long after the radiotherapy has been concluded.

Another study showed that rectal bleeding occurred in between 3 and 15 percent of radiotherapy patients, and persisted for more than six months in 3 percent of these cases. Pernicious diarrhea was diagnosed in about 2 percent, and cystitis with bleeding occurred in between 2 and 10 percent—a condition that lasted for more than six months in 3 percent of those same patients.

Bladder-neck strictures occurred in a little more than 1 percent of radiotherapy patients and incontinence in less than 1 percent, although the risk was higher in those patients who had already had TURPs.

Despite these side effects, about half of all prostate cancer patients who are given radiotherapy are permanently cured by it, whether it is administered with neo-adjuvant hormone therapy or without it. The results are best when the PSA drops quickly to zero or near-zero levels. The other half of these patients, however, develop a rising PSA after only two years, which means that their cancer, though not necessarily serious, may still be a threat.

If the PSA level increases in three consecutive counts after reaching its lowest point, the treatment is considered a failure. In one large study of more than 500 patients, 40 percent who had undergone radiotherapy lived for more than ten years after its completion.

Unfortunately, we don't have a precise way of determining how effective radiotherapy can be for any one patient, even when the Gleason Grade and the extent of the disease within the biopsy specimens are known. It is like using antibiotics without sensitivity testing; it may or may not work. It is very much hit and miss.

Less-established cancer treatments

It is human nature to speak less glowingly about treatments with which one has had little or no personal experience. I don't do perineal prostatectomies, which entail moving the gland through an incision made between the anus and the scrotum, and I seem to remember more negative remarks made about this procedure than I do positive ones. My feeling about cryoablation (intense freezing), hyperthermia (intense heating), and the use of laser beams and high-intensity focused ultrasound for the treatment of localized prostate cancer may also be prejudiced.

• Cryoablation is still being explored as a valid prostate cancer treatment in many centers, including one in London, Ontario, where my colleague and friend Dr. Joe Chin has won a reputation for being an established investigator. I know Dr. Chin as a competent, honest, and humble scholar; he sees a future in cryoablation and I trust his opinion. I also feel that this may take several more years to win widespread clinical acceptance. By and large, this is because most urologists have always felt that the transurethral cooling of the prostate will not attain the required temperature on the outside of the prostate, where the cancer is usually located.

Today, however, this treatment is not done through the urethra. As was pioneered back in the mid-1960s, between three and eight probes are injected into the prostate in the same way radioactive pellets are placed through the skin between the scrotum and rectum with ultrasound guidance. Liquid nitrogen is then passed into the probe until "ice balls" are seen on the monitor. A temperature between −350 degrees and −375 degrees Fahrenheit (−180° and −190°C) is achieved, and this can certainly cause cell death.

Furthermore, the difficulty with cryosurgery has always been how to achieve the proper temperature where it will count most without damaging adjacent tissue and organs. For this reason I suspect that it is enjoying only modest results—and with them came the danger that it may impair the rectum and the bladder.

- At the opposite end of the spectrum, hyperthermia uses microwave energy to attain a temperature of about 110 degrees Fahrenheit (43°C). Undoubtedly, when this heat is applied, prostate tissue is cooked. But, as hormone therapy is usually used in conjunction with hyperthermia, knowing how much cancer is killed with hyperthermia alone is difficult to ascertain.

In Toronto, Dr. John Trachtenberg, one of my former students who is now enjoying an international reputation as a prostate cancer scientist, has been exploring hyperthermia that uses temperatures considerably higher than 110 degrees

Fahrenheit (43°C), but only on selected patients in whom hormone therapy has failed. He tells me that he has been impressed with what the microwave can do.

- Temperatures are considerably hotter with laser therapy. This transforms light into heat so that a temperature of more than 140 degrees Fahrenheit (60°C) is attained for a few seconds. By this method, tissue is destroyed—including that harboring cancer cells—but the demarcation line between what needs to be zapped and what needs to be spared from this onslaught is fuzzy and inexact.

- Even higher temperatures—210 degrees Fahrenheit (100°C)—are achieved with high-intensity focused ultrasound through probes in the rectum. But this is only attained where the beams, fired into the prostate from different angles, converge. Clinical studies are just beginning on this modality of treatment, but on a theoretical level, it seems promising.

The search for the *absolute* treatment for prostate cancer continues. What we do know is that when it is diagnosed early, it is more effectively dealt with by surgery than by anything else. Studies show that more patients are alive and well fifteen years after a radical prostatectomy than they are with radiotherapy. When radiotherapy is administered with hormonal therapy, however, the results may be the same as surgery.

Some people might look at these results with suspicion, claiming that they are askew, that urologists may have operated only on the younger, healthier men, the "good" patients, and referred the older, sicker ones (the "bad" patients) for radiotherapy so as to be able to boast more surgical successes. Both surgical and radiotherapy results, however, are improving all the time. Sometimes the choice for the patient is obvious, as when he is unfit for surgery, very elderly, or morbidly obese.

Often, the choice for or against surgery is made after much homework and deliberation. I try to steer my younger patients with early but aggressive tumors toward it, but I generally steer men who are over seventy-two years old, and those with extensive local disease, toward radiotherapy. So, while the palliative option is hormone treatment, the curative options are very definitely radiotherapy—or surgery.

15. Prostate cancer: Preparing for surgery

The very best candidates for radical prostatectomies are men under sixty-five with no other health problems, or those over this age who have good family medical histories of longevity. They are most likely to have early confined prostate cancer, staged as a T1c or a T2a.

- T1c describes a situation wherein there was nothing suspicious on the rectal examination, but an elevated PSA reading led to a transrectal ultrasound and an ultrasound-guided biopsy.
- T2a disease is one that has demonstrated a suspicious nodule in the prostate on rectal examination. While the PSA could be normal, it is more likely to be slightly elevated.

A bone scan on a prospective radical prostatectomy patient will seldom be necessary because this operation seeks only to treat early disease, not that which has spread. A radical prostatectomy, then, is always done with a complete cancer cure in mind. On rare occasions, though, it may be used to control locally advanced cancer.

Let me introduce the preparation for this operation with a philosophical aside. From time to time, fundamental shifts occur in the way medicine is practiced. The introduction of antiseptic measures in hospitals and operating rooms was revolutionary, and as much a shift in medicine as the advent of antibiotics. Blood transfusions and anticoagulants may also qualify as being part of a major shift in the broad scope of medical science. The displacement of long surgical incisions by puncture holes for procedures with scopes and cameras may represent another innovation.

The catchphrases of the day, however, are "evidence-based medicine" and "patient participation in the decision-making process." This means that when it comes to a serious issue—like prostate cancer—patients are expected to do their homework before deciding on what course of action should be taken so that doctors may not impose one on unsuspecting patients.

Computer-literate patients surf the Internet to gather information that will help them make a decision. Curiously, people seem to believe whatever they read on the Internet, even though there is often no editorial validation of what is posted. For this reason, many men who come to me with prostate cancer are ill-informed about what can, or should, be done for them. Some have read about improbable cures. It falls on me to set them straight.

Patients are prepared for a radical prostatectomy much as they are for any other major procedure, but there are considerations peculiar to this operation. Before the surgery is booked, I meet with the patient and/or his partner to lay out the pros and cons. The pros are usually quite simple. The moment I have removed the prostate gland, in a three-hour operation, the cancer is gone. The cons, however, are a little different and must be explained with frankness.

First, while incontinence is no longer an issue in this kind of operation—surgeons have long since mastered the skill of what we call the "nerve-sparing" radical prostatectomy—there is still a 1 percent risk of it (treatable, though it is), as well as other nasty side effects, such as scarring at the neck of the bladder that may impede urination later by causing a blockage.

There are also risks of wound infections, lymphoceles, phlebitis, and pneumonia. I cannot remember when I last had a case of wound infection. Certainly, there has not been one in the past ten years, because wound-washing before closing the incision in this kind of operation has made a significant difference, and no resident doctor wants to be the one who is associated with the first case of infection to rear its ugly head in some time. I have, however, had four cases of lymphoceles. This, a collection of lymphatic fluid in the pelvic region, occurs when the lymphatic channels are not clipped during the surgery or because Heparin, a commonly used blood thinner, is used to reduce the risk of blood clots. It is not a serious complication, and most cases of it resolve themselves spontaneously or are relieved with needle drainage, but it is well worth avoiding as it can retard recovery.

Phlebitis—inflammation of the veins—can cause clots that may migrate to the lungs, causing what we call pulmonary embolisms. While the occurrence of this is quite rare as well, phlebitis itself is common and remains a painful condition for some weeks after the operation. To reduce the risk, hospitals issue patients white, knee-length support hose, and doctors routinely prescribe 5,000 units of Heparin at the start of surgery.

Another side effect is acute anemia, due to a considerable loss of blood during the surgery. To help deal with this during the operation, and after it, I discuss both the benefits and the disadvantages of a patient storing some of his own blood so it will be there if he needs it later.

A patient may donate up to 3 units (3 pints) during the four or five weeks prior to his surgery. I do not, however, encourage him to do this because it can weaken him at a time when he needs as much strength as he can muster to withstand the surgical assault. In any case, when blood is required, 3 units is usually not enough.

Instead, I encourage patients to determine if their insurance plans will cover the cost of Eprex (erythropoietin), a genetically engineered hormone that stimulates the production of red blood cells. I have adopted the American urologist Herbert Lepor's scheme. He gave 600 units per kilogram of the patient's weight—by injection—two weeks before surgery, with a further 300 units per kilogram if the hematocrit (the proportion of red cells in the blood) is less than 46 percent just one week before.

To anticipate the probable removal of one of the two bladder-control muscles during surgery, the patient is taught how to do a simple exercise—the Kegel exercise—which is designed to strengthen the muscle that remains. Instruction on how to do this exercise properly is provided by the nurse on the patient's preop visit, and reinforced either by myself or by a resident whenever the opportunity arises.

The exercise entails contracting the same muscles one would use to stop the urine in midstream, several times per hour. When it is properly achieved, the buttocks are squeezed together, and the rectum is made to contract.

In my early days, I did not insist that patients learn the Kegel exercise before the operation, and it is difficult to learn it immediately afterward because it can be painful. Yet it is important. Whenever I tell my students this, I cannot help but recall one patient who was totally incontinent. His idea of the Kegel exercise was to strain every drop of urine from his bladder every few minutes. Once he understood he had to contract exactly the opposite muscle, he rapidly gained control and his wetting stopped.

By far the most disturbing and overriding effect of the radical prostatectomy is erectile dysfunction, which is permanent in 75 percent of cases. Many men recover their potency after a few months, while others say it takes up to two years. Still more, however, are unable to regain their potency at all.

It is not always easy for a urologist to tell a once-virile man that his natural sex life may come to an end with his surgery, but doctors the world over are forever mindful of Dr. Walsh's admonition that the sole purpose of a radical prostatectomy is to cure cancer, not to preserve potency.

With at least 500 radical prostatectomies behind me—and having taught two generations of urology residents how to do them for themselves—I disagree with some of my American colleagues who maintain that the procedure should be done only by a select few. It is, of course, one of the more difficult operations for the trainee to do, and for this reason I always stress that attention to detail goes a long way toward reducing the risk of complications. I honestly believe I am helping a new breed of urologist master this procedure.

I am heartened, too, to know that in many of the operations I have performed, the side effects—permanent or otherwise—have been relatively few indeed.

Walking testimony of this was a slightly overweight businessman of sixty who was healthy despite having had a triple coronary bypass operation two years before consulting me with prostate problems. He had a PSA reading of 8.8, which led automatically to an ultrasound-guided biopsy. This, in turn, showed a Gleason Grade 6 tumor, which now occupied much of the left apex of his prostate.

This man, who had already visited several centers in the United States and had read all manner of prostate literature on the Internet, came to see me reluctantly upon the insistence of a friend. He gave me a few minutes to study his documents and then barked, "Are you the very best surgeon in the world for this operation?"

"As a matter of fact, I am," I replied, "but I expect every other surgeon who does this operation to be able to say the same thing."

"Very clever answer," the businessman replied. "I'll get back to you. I have a young wife, you know, and there are certain expectations."

I did the radical prostatectomy a few weeks later, and, fortunately for me—and for the patient—he is dry (incontinence-free) and potent, and his PSA readings are zero.

Another man was far less suspicious when he came to me with a Gleason Grade 4 cancer that had been found during an ultrasound-guided biopsy. Watchful waiting was suggested by a number of urologists he'd consulted, and I agreed with this.

Meanwhile, the man's PSA of 7.2 continued to climb slowly, and as it did, we did another biopsy. Now the Gleason Grade was 8, and I suggested radiotherapy. The patient, however, rejected the idea out of hand, considering himself both young enough and fit enough for a radical prostatectomy.

I was persuaded to carry out this operation two years after having first met this man, and I am happy to report that he is dry with a PSA of zero, and can function quite well in the bedroom for a seventy-four-year-old man—with Viagra! He has since suggested that I might consider doing radical prostatectomies more often on men of his age.

The suggestion that I may have been the very best surgeon for this operation may seem extraordinarily arrogant, but it is intended to reflect the kind of confidence every doctor should possess. During a court appearance, the renowned American cardiovascular specialist Dr. Denton Cooley once claimed he was the best surgeon in the world.

"How can you make such a claim?" asked the judge.

"Under oath," Cooley replied.

I would like to have been under oath when I verified that one man actually benefited from his prostatectomy, if you can believe it! In his native St. Vincent, in the West Indies, early prostate cancer was diagnosed, and he sought me out in Canada to perform his operation. The surgery itself, and the postoperative course, were uneventful. Far more memorable was this patient's remark when he saw me during a subsequent visit to my office.

"What did you do, doc?" he asked. "I mean, my erections are stronger now than they ever were before the operation!"

How it is done

In the twenty-four hours before his surgery, the patient is prepared for the operating theater. His pubic hair is removed, and he undergoes a mechanical bowel clean-out with laxatives and enemas. This can be done at home on the evening prior to surgery, or at the hospital in the hours preceding it.

The anesthesiologist is the first person to prepare the patient in the operating room. He or she places a small plastic tube through the shaft of a needle between the lumbar-region vertebrae, as is done for a spinal anesthetic. In reality, however, this is not a "spinal" at all. The tube is actually in the space outside the spinal canal; this tubing will be kept in place until a day or two after surgery in case it is needed for the administration of pain medications.

An intravenous line will be started in the arm in the operating room, and another needle will be placed in the wrist artery (radial artery) to monitor oxygen levels in the blood during the operation. The patient will be put to sleep with a drug that is fed into the intravenous line, and, subsequently, a tube (endotracheal) will be slipped down his throat into the trachea, or windpipe, to prevent him from swallowing his tongue.

As in the case of a simple retropubic prostatectomy, sometimes done for an enlarged prostate, a plastic tube will also be placed in the jugular. The height of the blood level in this tube monitors the blood volume. Now, the patient is ready for me—the surgeon.

16. Prostate cancer: The radical prostatectomy

Most radical prostatectomies done today seek to spare those nerves that are needed to maintain sexual function—a procedure first introduced by Dr. Walsh at Johns Hopkins in 1982, which has been modified in many minor ways since. What is known as the "nerve-sparing" prostatectomy is still considered one of the most difficult operations for the urology resident to master.

Urologists, whose reputations and notoriety are in some measure based on this operation, compound the problem by insisting that patients seek out only those surgeons who have performed it more than 100 times. If, however, we permit a training urologist only to open and close the abdominal incision required for this operation, rather than do the other work so vital to excise the gland (as some of my American colleagues would have it), how will we train him or her to do the complete operation alone?

This attitude of not allowing residents to do very much in the operating theater is understandable in a litigious society like the United States, but I wonder how the next generations of surgeons can ever be developed unless they are given diverse on-the-job experience. Thus, at the Royal Victoria Hospital, a resident who has assisted me in a procedure once—whether it be a radical prostatectomy or a TURP—is expected to be able to do it next time around with me as the coach.

I enjoy the challenge of this operation. As I scrub up for it with my assistant, usually a senior resident, we discuss the details of the patient's history, and, more precisely, the location and extent of his tumor. We do this because we want to know just how complex the operation may turn out to be.

If the patient's PSA is under 10 and his Gleason Grade is under 6, we know we will be embarking upon a fairly routine radical prostatectomy, with almost no complications. If, however, these numbers are higher, we can expect something different.

We will have to anticipate, for example—though we are not always correct—that the cancer may already have spread into the lymph nodes. In any case, a patient who has a Gleason Grade 7 or higher and a PSA above 10 routinely undergoes what we call a lymph node dissection. This means that we will have to cut out the obturator nodes, which are deep in the pelvis, and send them to the pathologist for a frozen-section examination for cancer before deciding whether or not to proceed with the prostatectomy.

Whatever has to be done, as the anesthesiology team finishes its preliminary work, my resident positions the patient supine for this operation. It is also important for him to see that the patient lies with the break in the operating table in line with his pubic bone. This is so that when the table is tented up, the patient will be lying with his pelvic region elevated.

This exaggerated extension of the abdomen is particularly useful for me when I am operating on patients who are overweight. This position may later cause some back pain, but that has not been my general experience. Nor have I found separating the legs either necessary or useful.

When this has been done, and when the anesthesiologist and an assistant are preparing for the next phase of their work, I enter the theater, adjust the overhead lighting and the height of the operating table, and begin my part of the procedure.

First, I paint and drape the patient and insert a Foley catheter so his bladder will remain empty throughout the entire operation. Now I make the one and only skin incision—in a straight line from the navel down to the pubic bone.

Beneath the skin there is a lot of fat, and underneath that, a thick, white tendinous layer that covers the midline muscles. When this sheath is cauterized open, with an electrical current to minimize bleeding, the midline recti muscles can be pulled apart, and held in position by adjustable retractors that are fixed to the operating table.

Having pushed the fat aside, I can see both the artery and the vein that run from the abdomen to the legs. These are not important to the work I will routinely do, except that they define the outer margins of my operating field. The deflated bladder marks the top, and the pubic bone the bottom. The area in which I actually cut out the prostate gland, however, and rejoin the urethra to the bladder, is about the size of my two hands when they are held side by side.

If I know that I must remove the obturator nodes for frozen-section examination, I do this at this time—and wait for the pathologist's report. Usually, the results are returned from the lab to the theater within about fifteen minutes, so the delay in the prostatectomy is never very long.

Once I know that the nodes are cancer-free, I can continue with the operation. If, however, they are positive, I see no point—or advantage—in removing the patient's prostate gland and making him suffer unnecessarily. Sometimes, he and I will have agreed beforehand: If the nodes are only minimally involved, I will proceed with the prostatectomy; if extensive cancer is found in the nodes, I will remove his testicles under the same anesthetic.

If no such agreement has been made, I simply close the incision, and the resident and I start thinking about which alternatives we must turn to.

When the actual removal of the prostate is in order, the operation is begun carefully. I mop away a collection of fatty tissue from each side of the gland to find a thin, almost transparent, membrane of tissue called the endopelvic fascia. I must cut into this in order to feel—with my gloved fingers—the side walls of the gland from the base of the bladder to the beginning of the urethra.

Now I turn my attention to a mass of fat and blood vessels that are on top of the prostate at its junction with the urethra. When most of this has been removed, again by electrocautery "cooking," I apply downward pressure to the prostate to expose two tendons that run from the pubic bone. These are known as the puboprostatic ligaments, and their sole job is to keep the gland in position.

Cutting them away to free the prostate is not always easy. Beneath these ligaments, and on either side, are huge veins. If the ligaments are not carefully snipped, and the veins are incised in error, there can be profuse bleeding.

Once I have cut these ligaments as close as possible to the pubic bone, I can depress the gland toward the rectum even more, this time exposing an area large enough for me to tie off the veins. This is one of the trickiest stages of the entire operation because an error in the next step means a very bloody case, indeed.

I slide my finger along the side of the prostate, just beyond the apex, and feel the top of the urethra where it contains the catheter. I then pass long-beaked MacDougal forceps just above the urethra from right to left, or from left to right. A strong suture is fed into the bite of the forceps and pulled through the mass of tissue that contains those blood vessels to tie them off tightly. I must now anchor this stitch with a bite into the same tissue so that it will not slip off.

When the long-beaked forceps are passed into the same aperture, and a cut is made above it, the prostate will have been freed from the large veins in front of it. The junction of the prostate and the urethra can now be cleanly dissected—in a bloodless field. For the moment, however, I am still preparing the way.

I now lift the urethra with the forceps, like picking up a strand of spaghetti with tongs, so I can get an instrument around it. Because there has been no adequate tool for this intricate maneuver, I have had to make one for myself. One day, I went to the hospital machine shop with a pair of tongs that we typically use to hold tissue without damaging it (a Babcock clamp) and asked a machinist to adapt them into something resembling carpenter's pincers. I ensured, however, that the bowed tips of these "pincers" were blunt so that when I used them to lift the urethra they did the job without bruising.

Back to the operation: I slip the same long-beaked forceps underneath these adapted forceps as they hold up the urethra, staying very close to it. This is so I will not damage those nerves that are responsible for the patient's erection. A small tape, the kind used to tie off the umbilical cord in a newborn, is then fed into the forceps and passed under the urethra so I can lift it sufficiently to be able to cut it open as close to the prostate as possible—without damaging the sphincter this time, the valve that prevents the urine from leaking.

The way is now free for me to make an incision across the top of the urethra at the base of the prostate, rather than amputate it completely. If I did this prematurely, there would be a danger that the urethra might retract into the penis and complicate the operation. So, at this point, I place two strong sutures—at ten o'clock and two o'clock—in the half-cut urethra so that they are nicely in place when I *do* eventually amputate it, and when I finally need to join it directly to the bladder after the prostate has been removed. With one careful cut, I then complete the amputation.

With strong traction on the catheter, which is still running through the prostate into the bladder, I move to the next step. I free the gland on each side toward the bladder. This is another tricky part. As I go along the outer side walls of the prostate, there again looms the danger of damaging those same erectile nerves, so I must continue to be cautious.

Here, for the next step of the nerve-sparing radical prostatectomy, I introduce a second instrument I have adapted for it. This is used to free the gland from its densely adherent connective tissue and blood vessels, and branches of the same nerves. The dissection must be razor-sharp rather than blunt, and this means I have to cut rather than tease away. When I cut, I must have complete control of the blood vessels before any incision is made.

The instrument I adapted is a curve-shaped set of forceps that carry a silk thread in a V-shaped groove on the outside. I use this instrument, which I had made by a physicist friend (Dr. Morrel Bachynski of MPB Industries, a Montreal fiber-optics company), to traverse the outer contour of the gland. The thread is used to tie off all that dense tissue before I make the final cut to release the gland from its moorings just below the bladder. In effect, I am freeing the prostate while preparing to cut it off, and making sure that I don't damage nerves or cause unnecessary bleeding.

After a Radical Prostatectomy

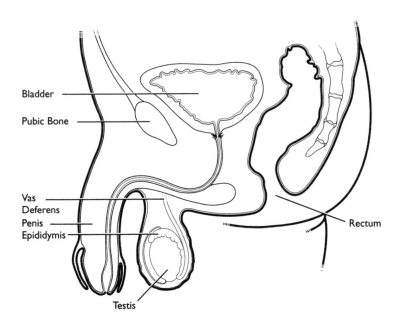

Bladder

Pubic Bone

Vas
Deferens

Penis

Epididymis

Rectum

Testis

Once the gland has been isolated, I can "hinge" it up, or flip it back, and cut into a lining known as "Denonvillier's fascia." This exposes both the seminal vesicles and the vas deferens, which carry the spermatozoa from the testicles. In a relatively simple part of the operation, the seminal vesicles are dissected out, and the vas is clipped.

Now the prostate is held only by the bladder neck, and I cut it away little by little, holding it like a dead bloom about to be chopped from its stem. If the preparation is done completely—and meticulously—removing the prostate from the bladder neck is easy.

The gland may now be out, but the next step is to reconstitute that section of the urinary tract. This, too, is a relatively simple job. If the operation has been done carefully thus far, the bladder neck will not have been damaged, and the aperture will, ideally, be about the thickness of my index finger. Years ago, before this "bladder-neck preserving" technique was developed, the aperture was three fingers wide, and this is why a lot of men were rendered incontinent for a much longer period after their surgery than they are today. Thankfully, this worry has been largely eliminated.

The neck of the bladder is rejoined to the urethra neatly, lining to lining, to avoid another possible side effect, a poor urine flow due to scarring. For this part of the operation, I use only four stitches, two of which, remember, were already put in place before the gland was excised. Stitches in the four o'clock and eight o'clock positions are now added. All four of these are now ready to join the urethra with the bladder neck. Before securing them tightly to make a proper joint, I ask for the operating table to be flattened. This ensures that the stitches will not pull out when they are tied.

At this point, the resident and I insert a small pipe that prevents any urine that may leak from the joint from accumulating around the wound, and we close the incision. The patient is then taken to the Intensive Care Unit for a few hours, where the jugular tube is usually removed. After nurses are satisfied that his heart is functioning properly, and that his blood pressure is adequate, he is wheeled to his room, where he typically begins a four- or five-day recovery period.

During this time the drainage tube is taken out and the patient is kept pain-free, given antibiotics, and subjected to daily blood tests that are designed to measure kidney function and levels of anemia. As he strengthens, his intravenous and epidural lines are removed, and the nurses encourage him to do breathing exercises to prevent pneumonia and to walk as much as possible to avoid phlebitis.

A few days after going home, the patient's skin clips—I don't use stitches on the skin incision—are removed by a visiting nurse. The Foley catheter, however, remains in place for a full two weeks, until the wound has healed sufficiently well to permit normal urination.

Although any nurse can remove a catheter, I usually like to do it myself following this kind of surgery—after using it to fill the patient's bladder. I want to see if he can urinate properly and stop his flow in midstream. Even though he may be able to urinate quite well, and cease urination on command, he is usually not fully continent right away.

One patient may be "dry" from the beginning while another may not, remaining incontinent for several weeks or months. In this case, more Kegel exercises will be needed to help him gain total control, and I want to ensure that he knows this as soon after his radical prostatectomy as possible.

Two months after his prostatectomy, the patient must return to the hospital for a PSA blood test that will tell me if it has been successful. Every six months thereafter, for the rest of his life, he will need another one—this time to tell me if he requires further treatment.

I cannot end this account of what is involved in the nerve-sparing radical prostatectomy without referring again to a patient or two. One of them came to see me for a routine checkup, and, during this brief visit, I detected a little asymmetry and an area of extra firmness in his prostate's left lobe. An ultrasound-guided biopsy later revealed that he had a Gleason Grade 7 cancer.

Because this man was only fifty-two and had a PSA of a mere 2.2, I felt he was an excellent candidate for a radical prostatectomy. In fact, I thought that his good health and relative youth made this the *absolute* treatment of choice. The patient, however, had other ideas, largely because he wanted as little time off from his work as an electronic company's financial officer as possible. He also thought that, having recently been widowed, he might one day meet another woman and need to reactivate his sex life.

"You realize," I told him, "that if you have radiotherapy first and it fails, surgery afterward is not an option. Not at all."

"Oh, why?" the man asked.

"Because radiotherapy turns the surrounding area into concrete," I explained, "and this makes removing the prostate virtually impossible."

"Really?"

"It would be like chipping away at stone to remove your cancer," I said, "yet if you had surgery first then needed radiotherapy afterward, it would be a perfectly good backup treatment, and one that would be likely to work."

The outcome of our discussions was that the patient would seek other opinions, which I encouraged.

First, he went to Boston, where conformal radiotherapy was advised by a radiotherapist, and where surgery was suggested by a surgeon. He finally decided on brachytherapy as the treatment least likely to interfere with his business commitments, and one that had a good chance of preserving his potency.

This took him to Seattle, where the radioactive iodine was placed by my friend Dr. Haakon Radge, one of the pioneers in this field, and within only a matter of days, the patient was back at work and happy with his choice. I fear, however, that it is too early for us to know what the final outcome will be. He must certainly be carefully monitored for as long as he is alive.

Contrast him, if you will, with a colleague physician—coincidentally also fifty-two—who came to see me for his annual prostate examination because his regular urologist was away. This man had a long-standing history of chronic prostatitis, which acted up from time to time, causing him a lot of discomfort. His PSA had been elevated to between 7.6 and 8.2 for several years, but this had been attributed to his prostatitis.

I recommended an ultrasound and biopsy for peace of mind, if nothing else. On examining the gland with my finger, I did not suspect cancer at all. In the report following an ultrasound-guided biopsy, however, cancer was detected in three of the six needles. It was a shock not only to the patient, but to me as well.

He, like most of the men who come to see me, took my advice when I suggested surgery. Now, three years after it, his PSA is almost zero (0.03), his potency is intact, and he is fully continent. Still, like a lot of men who have had radical prostatectomies and have many years of good living ahead of them, he tells me that he has a "panic attack" whenever it is time for another blood test.

A lot of my patients react in much the same way. I always feel, however, that it is also part of a urologist's job to remind them that surgery is nearly always a cure for early prostate cancer. Before PSA testing was developed, we had no way of knowing when prostate cancer had occurred or recurred. Now that we have PSA testing, we are presented with a double-edged sword—whether to know when cancer lurks or live blissfully in ignorance of its presence.

I think, if I were still relatively young, that I would prefer the devil I know to the devil who is still a stranger.

17. Prostate cancer: Incontinence and impotence

Without a doubt, incontinence and impotence are the two most dreaded side effects that may follow treatment for prostate cancer. Even with the best care in the world, with the best surgical hands, men usually suffer either or both of these afflictions, if only temporarily. Nonetheless, they are disconcerting disorders, and they are constantly on the minds of nearly all patients as they begin the long, seemingly endless path to recovery.

Here is the basic information:

- When administered alone, hormone treatment, which is usually reserved for men with advanced cancer, does not cause incontinence. Eventually, however, it will cause impotence, but this usually occurs at a time when a man will have lost all desire for sex. After all, the very nature of the treatment—to decrease testosterone levels—inhibits sexual desire in a matter of months.

- Radiotherapy carries virtually no risk of incontinence, though there are recorded cases, but there is up to a 50 percent chance of impotence.

- A radical prostatectomy carries a 1 percent chance of total incontinence and up to a 30 percent chance of mild incontinence. The impotence rate can vary from 30 to 80 percent.

As a rule, surgeons report better results about urinary control and erectile dysfunction when they talk directly to patients than do independent investigators seeking this information independently in questionnaires. I suspect this is because patients are less critical when discussing their posttreatment problems with their urologists than they are when they can hide behind the anonymity of a survey.

At any rate, incontinence and impotence are such psychologically crippling complications of prostate cancer that they must be fully addressed here.

Incontinence

Patients invariably ask, "Can anything be done for my incontinence? After all, it was caused by my surgery. When I've fully recovered from what you did inside me, will my incontinence stop automatically? Will I have to wear a diaper forever, doctor?"

If these questions imply that virtually all men suffer a little incontinence immediately after undergoing a radical prostatectomy, they should. I must be quick to add, however, that it usually lasts only a matter of days. We call it mild incontinence, and it occurs on coughing, straining, jumping, laughing, or rising from a sitting position.

When the operation is undertaken on a patient who has some degree of prostatic enlargement, the thickened bladder muscle that results from this is too much for the remaining sphincter to handle. The period of incontinence for such a man can be longer than for one who has not suffered bladder-muscle thickening. Whatever the degree of incontinence, a patient always benefits from those Kegel exercises because they strengthen his sphincter.

I find, however, that when the demands on a patient are too stringent, he doesn't do his exercises at all. Once-hourly contractions are all I ask him to aim for, and this can be quite effective. Of course, Kegel exercises are much better known to women. The diligent practice of them is routinely advised by gynecologists to treat and prevent stress incontinence after childbirth. The bonus for "Kegelling," as gynecologists call it, can actually be an enhanced sex life! That, however, is another matter.

While these exercises are very important for prostate cancer patients, there are medications that can help them, too. Some of these, like Ditropan (oxybutynin) or Detrol (tolterodine), work simply by instructing the nervous system to relax the bladder muscles. Other drugs, such as Urispas (flavoxate) or Valium (diazepam), relax the muscles directly.

I prescribe Ditropan in 5-milligram tablets, but because this drug causes "dry mouth" I ask patients to start by taking only half a pill a day for several days. Once their bodies are used to it, I increase the dosage to half a pill twice a day, eventually reaching one pill twice daily. I also advise them to have lemon drops, ice chips, candies, or gum on hand. Even then, the mucous membrane becomes so dry that a lot of patients don't like taking Ditropan. Fortunately, a slow-release version of the drug, with less dryness as a side effect, is expected in the near future.

Detrol is prescribed as a 2-milligram tablet twice a day. It is not quite as effective as Ditropan, but it doesn't dry the mouth quite as much, either. Thus, the dosage can be increased to optimize muscle relaxation. But this medication is expensive.

Urispas, meanwhile, is relatively free of all side effects but is effective only in a small percentage of patients. Valium is used more for its muscle-relaxing effect than its tranquilizing effect—although the latter can't hurt.

There are also medications that augment contractions of the sphincter muscle. Ironically, one of them is Sudafed (pseudoephedrine), which we know has caused a lot of problems for men with enlarged prostates, and which has mimicked the symptoms in others. This popular decongestant cold remedy, as well as the antidepressant Tofranil (imipramine), are the commonly used medications to help incontinence.

I prescribe Sudafed as a 60-milligram tablet in the morning, or 25 milligrams of Tofranil four times a day. Sometimes, I combine Sudafed or Tofranil with Detrol or Ditropan. If the patient's situation is improved by these medications, he is told to continue them for two months and then taper them off. It is usually not necessary to continue taking them for life.

When incontinence remains a major problem that has not responded to either exercise or medications, I carry out an internal examination with a cystoscope—another cystoscopy. During this I can see if the patient's sphincter is working. To find out, I ask him to make the sphincter contract. In other words, he must perform a Kegel exercise on the operating table.

With the scope in place I can see if the sphincter responds—or not. At that point, I want to ascertain if there is any scarring at the joint between the bladder and the urethra. If the sphincter—the "tap muscle"—is undamaged but weak, more Kegel sessions are advised, this time under the supervision of nurses or physiotherapists who use a monitor display to show the patient how well he is using the appropriate muscles. Reward, remember, reinforces effort.

If on cystoscopy the sphincter doesn't work, or if the examination does not render a clear-cut picture, urodynamic tests are done. In these video urodynamics the bladder is filled through a catheter with a dye that will show up on X-ray. If the bladder contracts a number of times with what we call uninhibited contractions as it is being filled, it is deemed to be overactive, in which case the incontinence should eventually be helped by Ditropan or Detrol. On the other hand, a persistent "funnel" appearance at the bladder neck signifies sphincter incompetence or sphincter damage. This diagnosis is reinforced when the patient is asked to "strain down" as if to force a bowel movement. A urine leak with a bladder pressure reading of less than 40 centimeters indicates a severely damaged sphincter.

Such a patient may have to accept any one of the following:
- a lifetime of adult diapers
- a permanent catheter
- a urine-collection device worn externally
- injections of an animal protein substance to augment the sphincter
- a penile Cunningham clamp
- the installation of an artificial sphincter

Some patients cope quite well with diapers and the occasional use of a Cunningham clamp. This, a padded "clothespin" device, effectively pinches the shaft of the penis closed to shut off the flow. The patient releases the clamp when he feels his bladder is full and allows the urine to pour out.

Other patients prefer a condom-like drainage device. The tip of the "condom" is connected to an open tube that channels urine into a leg bag. Essentially, the catheter does a similar job, except that it is interior while the condom device is exterior and, therefore, will not expose the patient to as many urine infections.

The injection of materials to augment the sphincter—by increasing resistance to urine that has collected in the bladder—is rather like adding a new washer to a leaky faucet. Teflon, silicone, and various body fats have all been tried, with varying degrees of success. Teflon and silicone can migrate to the lungs and cause other problems, while fat cells are too quickly absorbed into the body to do any good.

A protein product called bovine collagen, which is made from cows, has been used successfully. To insert it, a cystoscope is passed directly into the bladder through the skin in the lower abdomen. I can actually watch the liquid collagen being injected under the lining around the bladder and can ensure that it reaches the right place in the right quantity for maximum effectiveness.

The results of this simple procedure have been heartening. Improved urine control has been reported in 70 percent of men who have undergone it. When the same injection is tried through the penis, though, it is much less successful because we can't get the "washer" to sit correctly.

When all else has failed, a patient who does not want to wear a catheter, or diapers, or a clumsy collection device will need to be fitted with an artificial sphincter. This is simple in concept but, I'm afraid to tell you, quite crude in application.

The most common such device used today is called the AMS 800, distributed by Pfizer. It is something like a miniature of the cuff that a nurse wraps around your upper arm when he or she wants to take your blood pressure. This bandage-like device, which measures about an inch (2.5 cm) wide, has three pressure settings—between 50 and 60 centimeters, between 61 and 70 centimeters, and between 71 and 80 centimeters—and can be adjusted according to the need.

Basically, an artificial sphincter is wrapped around the urethra and filled with water instead of air. A squeeze-pump inserted into the scrotum moves this water from one compartment into another. As it does so, it either inflates the cuff, thus compressing the urethra to close it, or releases that pressure and opens the urethra to allow the urine to flow out.

It is, however, less than perfect. In 10 percent of cases, the pressure required to trap the urine causes the cuff to eat into the urethra. In this event, it must be quickly removed.

Sometimes it may be safely reinstalled, but on other occasions, if the urethra is too badly damaged, it shouldn't be. If we were to install an artificial sphincter on a scarred, bruised, or torn urethra, we would create more serious medical problems. Urine might leak from the area of the cuff and break through to the skin at the base of the penis, causing all manner of tissue infections.

What needs to be developed is an artificial sphincter that would work under much lower cuff pressure—a device that would be installed at the base of the bladder and *inside* the urethral wall. This might simply work by being inflated or expanded to trap the urine and deflated to let it flow again. It would not need to do this by squeezing the urethra and damaging it. What I'm suggesting is a little contraption that could be made to "block" the urine with the simple squeeze of a pump, then be able to "unblock" it to allow the bladder to empty.

Erectile dysfunction

Impotence after a radical prostatectomy or radiotherapy is the subject of much discussion and controversy in urological circles. The problem is how to interpret the statistics. For example, a surgeon who claims that all his patients are fully potent after having performed radical prostatectomies on them cannot possibly be telling the truth. For one, the nature of the surgery nearly always impairs erectile nerves. For two, his patients did not belong to a fully potent sector of society in the first place, let alone a sexually active one.

Published statistical evidence—gathered for a study by the famed sexologists William Masters and Virginia Johnson—shows that as many as one-third of men over sixty are not sexually active, and that more than half of all men over seventy aren't either. This doesn't mean that these men *cannot* have sex because they cannot get an erection. It does, however, suggest that at the time of their treatment, and the follow-up to it, their erectile ability was not uppermost in their minds. Consequently, they could not provide valuable input to any kind of study on impotence.

Actually, assessments of potency before or after prostate cancer treatment are seldom made, or, if they are, they are not made precisely. This may be because sexual function seems inconsequential at a time when cancer is the major concern. So, if a man has a weak erection prior to surgery, and no erection after it, he might want to blame his surgeon—rather than the ravages of time.

Nevertheless, erectile difficulties remain intimately associated with radiotherapy and radical prostate surgery.

The 50 percent of patients who are *not* rendered impotent after radiotherapy will report penises that are shorter and thinner but say there is no change in their libido or sexual enjoyment. Prolonged radiotherapy quite often injures blood vessels, and this is doubtless why the penis may shrink by an inch (2.5 cm) or so.

Unfortunately, surgery can also shrink a penis and render a patient totally impotent, even when a nerve-sparing procedure has been meticulously followed. (Good erections are much more likely to be preserved in younger men than they are in older ones.) It is not clear whether a total loss of potency is due to inadvertent injury to the neurovascular bundles—those nerves that are found on each side of the prostate gland—or because of other factors. More certain is that most surgeons will admit to not really knowing if they have damaged the erectile nerves.

This explains why I tell each prostatectomy patient, after he has been returned to the ward, "Your operation went well, and you should have no problem with urine control. I'm not sure about the erection, though. We'll have to wait and see."

The power of Viagra

When the restoration of erection is important to a patient, a number of therapeutic measures can be considered. For most men, Viagra (sildenafil) will be the first and simplest thing to try. There is no question that Viagra has caused a sensation around the world, and millions of men have tried it. The stampede to the corner drugstore after its March 1998 release in the United States has been unmatched in the case of any other medications.

This wonderful drug, manufactured by Pfizer, works best on patients who are not totally impotent, but it is nonetheless worth giving to those who are.

Even older men are aided by Viagra. One such patient was ninety years old, if you can believe it, and had been a visitor to my office for some twenty-five years. Many of his friends had passed on, some from prostate cancer, and many others had had TURPs, radical prostatectomies, hormone treatments, radiation treatments, and a combination of them all. My patient was lucky, though. He was still alive.

I suspect he came regularly for his annual prostate examination simply to hear me say, "You have the gland of a twenty-five-year-old!" I might not have been wrong.

One day, as he was about to depart my office, he suddenly stopped in the doorway, jerked back his head, and asked, "Is there any reason why I can't try Viagra, doc?"

I was taken aback at first, but decided to discuss the matter. "You don't take pills for a weak heart," I said. "You don't even take blood pressure pills. You're in excellent health! So there is no reason why you can't try Viagra."

"Really?"

"But as you may know," I continued, "Viagra works only when you're in the mood—and when you have a willing and eager partner."

I was clearly making an assumption I had no right to make.

"But, doc," the patient added, "it's my wife who asked me to ask you."

I gave him his prescription and instructed him to take the pill, with lots of water on an empty stomach, one hour before sex.

Patients who suffer erectile dysfunction after prostate cancer treatment may choose to accept their disabilities. Many men I see have done exactly this—often to the relief of their partners who are simply glad to know that their partners are alive.

Many other patients, though, are not willing to accept the demise of their sex lives, and they equate this with a loss of potency. The two are not the same thing, however, as other patients so often tell me. Men with minimal erections still engage in enjoyable sexual activities, and they tell me exactly what these are. Some of these same men admit that their erectile dysfunctions have somehow brought them closer to their partners, or that their partners have shown unsurpassed compassion and understanding for their problems.

Suffice it to say that when an erection is particularly important to a patient, and he can't get one, I start him on Viagra. It is a first-line treatment. There is, however, one proviso: The pill alone is not enough. As I told that ninety-year-old man, atmosphere, mood, and the cooperation of a sex partner is vital for Viagra to work.

There are, however, exceptions to who should or should not take Viagra. Men who are on medications for angina definitely must *not* take it. Patients on heavy doses of antihypertensive drugs can take Viagra, but they are often afraid to do so. As an experiment, I ask them to try a 25-milligram dose before sex and take note of its effectiveness. Such a small amount of this drug is unlikely to create an erection, but neither is it likely to cause complications. If there are no adverse effects, I may feel confident in doubling the dose, and this is much more likely to succeed.

When I get requests for Viagra from men who are blue in the face after having walked a mere 10 yards (9 meters), I turn them down.

We must be careful with Viagra—very careful. So, if a well-meaning friend offers you a tablet or two, you should decline. Almost everyone has heard of Viagra-related deaths, and it is a real problem.

So far, about 200 men around the world may have died from causes associated with the use of Viagra. What is not clear is how many of them died from the drug itself, and how many from the exertion of sexual intercourse. I point out to worried patients that not one fatality occurred during the drug's initial worldwide trials on literally tens of thousands of men, and that 200 deaths do not seem overwhelming when more than a hundred people die annually from herbal preparations.

Nor were there any serious problems encountered when McGill University's Department of Urology tested Viagra as part of a widespread study of more than 4,000 impotent men. One volunteer, an engineer, complained of bad headaches when he took Viagra. Headaches, facial flashes, and short-lived changes in color perception (everything looked a little blue, it seemed) were other recognized side effects.

"Do you want to come off the trial?" the engineer was asked.

"No way!" he responded.

That was when I became certain a phenomenal product was about to be launched.

Usually when I prescribe Viagra, I do so in 100-milligram

tablets—then I ask the patient to take only half of one an hour or so before sex. Of course, I could prescribe him 50-milligram tablets, but, inexplicably, the cost is the same regardless of strength. So, because Viagra is expensive and may continue to be so for some time, I try to save my patients money.

Many patients are helped appreciably with the 50-milligram dosages, but others find 100-milligram tablets considerably more effective.

Two final points about Viagra: First, if it isn't successful on the first attempt, give it a chance. You may need to try it as many as six to eight times to benefit. Second, Viagra has been known to restore "youthful sexuality." So much so that, after having created one erection, it may generate two or three more within a thirty-six-hour period—without taking another pill. That's three for the price of one!

How Viagra was developed

The story of Viagra's rise to fame is worth relating. Scientists working at Pfizer's British branch were studying a new drug they hoped would lower blood pressure in people suffering from hypertension. Male volunteers who took the medication saw little change in their blood pressures but were reluctant to return unused pills. They noticed something they hadn't seen for some time—enhanced erections.

What a wonderful side effect!

The people at Pfizer agreed and began to study the drug for its possible effects on erectile dysfunction.

Was it all serendipitous? Could those volunteers have been wrong?

Actually, once the chemistry of male erections began to be understood, in the early 1990s, it was inevitable that a potency-promoting drug would be developed. The chemical molecule that the body manufactures to produce an erection is nitric oxide (NO). The postpubertal male releases this from the nerve endings within his penis the moment the things we come to associate with sexual appetite—sight, thought, and imagination—are stimulated, and when these are enhanced by smell or touch.

Nitric oxide works on an enzyme called "guanylate cyclase," which promotes the accumulation of cyclic guanosine monophosphate (cGMP). This compound reduces the amount of calcium inside the muscle cells of blood vessels within the penis, causing them to relax. The sponge-like blood vessels engorge with blood, then work like flap valves closing the exit door. The enclosed chamber fills to capacity, and the turgor, or rigidity, constitutes what we know as the erection.

After some time, the body releases another chemical product, called "phosphodiesterase," which breaks down the cGMP, reversing the process. The erection disappears.

Viagra works not by stimulating the erection, but by inactivating the chemical—phosphodiesterase—that brings an erection to an end. Thus, when the "inactivator" is inactivated, the penis is stimulated to engorge.

Voilà! The magic impotence pill—Viagra!

Phosphodiesterase itself is quite ubiquitous. It is in coffee, for instance. And, within this family of chemical compounds, a minor change in formulation makes one product more specific for one organ than another. Phosphodiesterase-5, for example, is specific to the penis, and sildenafil appears to inactivate this specific enzyme.

Viagra can cross-react with the other enzymes. For example, it can react with the enzyme associated with heart muscles, and this may be why cardiac problems can be caused by it. Furthermore, another form of this enzyme is found in the retina, which can account for occasional complaints of blurred vision, or that bluish tint men complained about during our study at McGill.

Pharmaceutical firms, like Pfizer, claim it costs $400 million to bring a new pill to market. For each drug developed, 10,000 may have been proposed. Of these, only ten to fifteen reach laboratory and safety testing. Six of these go for phase-one testing, in which healthy volunteers are used to test both the safety of the drug and its proper dosage. A further four go on to phase-two testing, in which the medication's effectiveness and side effects are studied.

Finally, one of these proposed medications makes the phase-three study. In this, the drug is tested for possible side effects on thousands of patients, usually worldwide. Based on the success of this, the drug proposal is then submitted for government approval.

The whole process of introducing one new drug takes between nine and sixteen years. Most countries, however, will not accept studies that were done abroad and end up repeating them for their own satisfaction. This is why a drug may appear in one country many years before it shows up in another.

Still, the manufacturing cost of the pill is minuscule, so the $10 to $15 charged for one Viagra pill in North America represents an enormous profit for Pfizer.

By becoming the first-line treatment for erectile dysfunction, Viagra has replaced Yohimbine and Trazodone, the only oral preparations that had any kind of positive results in the past. In time, Viagra will be challenged by other pills, some of which are already close to market.

They include:

- Spontane (apomorphine), which is made by TAP Pharmaceuticals. This drug, which is placed under the tongue about a half hour before sex, stimulates dopamine receptors in the brain and works best on psychologically based impotence. Its success rate is just over 50 percent, and its side effects appear to be relatively few. There can be nausea, but there are no other significant problems.

- Vasomax (phentolamine), which is made by Zonagen/Schering-Plough Pharmaceuticals. This is an oral version of a drug that is often used in combination with other preparations as a penile injection to induce an erection. The oral preparation has been hard to produce, and excess amounts are known to decrease blood pressure considerably. Nonetheless, a 40 percent success rate has been reported, and this is quite good.

- Other pills similar to Viagra, as well as a cream form of it, which are also under investigation—by several companies.

Without doubt, the development of pills to help such disorders as erectile dysfunction is a burgeoning field as medicine shifts its emphasis from diagnosis and treatment of serious maladies to the improvement of lifestyles. Obesity pills, intelligence pills, mood-changing pills, and longevity pills, not to mention herbs and vitamins, will become the order of the day. Pharmaceutical companies will spend millions developing these new preparations, and some of this money will be spent entirely on finding suitably attractive names for them—names that will ensure that they reach those corners of the market for which they are intended.

Viagra, for example, comes from a combination of "vigor," the essence of male sexual potency, and "Niagara," a name associated with the power of the famous falls. I have a suggestion for any competing product that may lay claim to promoting more orgasms.

How about Morgasm?

18. Erectile dysfunction: When Viagra doesn't work

As good as it is, Viagra doesn't always work and it is up to the urologist to decide what to do next. There are several options:

- a urethral suppository called MUSE
- a penile vacuum pump
- penile injections
- penile prostheses

The product popularly known as MUSE is a pellet derived from the drug alprostadil. It is deposited into the tip of the penis in an applicator. The patient voids to lubricate the passage, inserts the applicator, a tiny plastic tube about three-quarters of an inch (2 cm) long, and then presses a knob that releases the pellet.

Dosage comes in three strengths—250 micrograms, 500 micrograms, and 1,000 micrograms. Only the two stronger ones, however, are usually effective.

Once the pellet is in place, the penis is massaged between two hands, and, within twenty minutes, an erection should occur. At least about 60 percent of patients for whom Viagra has not worked attain an erection with MUSE. The downside is that it is more than double the price of Viagra.

When MUSE fails, a patient can still try what we call a vacuum pump, or he can inject a drug directly into the penis, or he can ask his urologist to insert a penile prosthesis.

The vacuum pump

The vacuum pump works according to the laws of physics, so it is not surprising that the device was invented by an auto mechanic and not a doctor! The full shaft of the penis is placed inside a plastic cylinder that has been fitted with tubing so that, when the device is held firmly against the body, all air can be sucked out of it.

As the air is withdrawn, equilibrium is sought and blood is pulled into the flaccid penis. When a sufficient erection is achieved, a rubber constriction ring is slipped off the cylinder onto the penis to retain the blood. The vacuum is then released, and the cylinder removed.

Not all patients are comfortable with this device, which has been around for many years. Some men find the vacuuming process too painful, and some find the constriction ring too uncomfortable. Other men, meanwhile, cannot attain sufficient rigidity. On the other hand, many patients are positively delighted with a contraption that does not add a chemical to their bodies.

There are several kinds of vacuum pumps. A cheap one can be bought in a sex shop for less than $100, while a more sophisticated one that is medically approved will cost between $300 and $1,000. The most expensive pumps create a vacuum with battery power, and this might be considered less tiresome at a time when a man's mind should be on other things.

Several patients have made their own erection-giving devices—by adapting bicycle pumps. The best one of these was made by a man who fashioned a $20-wine bottle pump, which is meant to evacuate the air from an unfinished bottle of champagne. All he needed to adapt this was a length of tubing and some strong glue. It worked.

A word of warning: Do not use your vacuum cleaner. One man who tried this stripped the skin off his penis.

Penile injections

Penile injections have become commonplace. Caverject (alprostadil), the same drug used in MUSE, is widely sold in fancy packages as 10- or 20-microgram doses.

The same drug, sold under a different name, comprises alprostadil in water, a solution that must be made by a pharmacist. Because it is in liquid form, it also has to be kept refrigerated. Caverject, however, is a combination of alprostadil (in powder form) and saline—and the solution can be mixed by the patient himself at the time of use. It does not therefore require any refrigeration.

When Caverject alone doesn't work satisfactorily, drugs called papaverine and phentolamine are added to make a mix. This combined preparation is widely known as "tri-mix."

Erectile dysfunction clinics across the world have taught countless men how to inject the drugs properly into the body of the penis. It is interesting to note that this entire enterprise was started by one man, Dr. G. S. Brindley of Britain, when he was himself long past middle age. Youth must be served, of course, but I wonder why we so commonly assume that an innovative measure cannot be the brainchild of a man older than forty.

There are side effects that should not be ignored. Priapism is one. This is defined as a painful, unrelenting erection that may last as long as six hours, and which, if left untreated, can lead to permanent penile damage and the inability to have erections in the future. This complication is generally treated urgently, however, by drawing some penile blood with another needle and injecting a vasoconstricting substance, like adrenalin. Of course this should only be done by a physician.

Although penile injections are known to work well, many patients try them and then stop using them. This is possibly due to fear of needles, a lack of spontaneity, or a combination of both. Furthermore, the side effects include pain upon injection, scarring of the lining of the erectile tissue (which can lead to penile curvature), and, though quite rare, an escape of the drug into the bloodstream, which can cause heart problems or lower blood pressure.

Penile prostheses

Viagra, MUSE, and the penile injections of vasoactive drugs have made the surgical insertion of penile prostheses less common today than they were a decade or so ago. Still, when Viagra, MUSE, pumps, and injections have failed to help a patient, and he still wishes to enjoy sexual activity, a prosthesis is the only answer.

The next question is: Which prosthesis should be installed?

When I treat an older patient who has suffered prostate cancer and who wants an uncomplicated prelude to any sexual activity, I usually recommend what we call the malleable prosthesis, rather than the inflatable one.

The inflatable prosthesis has too many moving parts that can go wrong—not to mention a pump that is inserted into the scrotum, and a reservoir of saline that is installed in front of the bladder. The malleable prosthesis, on the other hand, is one simple piece of tubing rather like a plumber's snake. It can be made to hinge up and down to assume any given shape, which it can hold.

Malleable Prosthesis

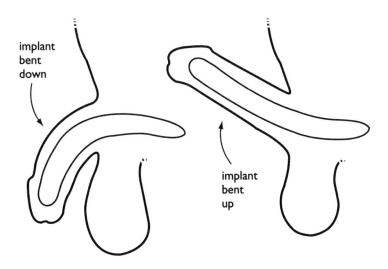

implant
bent
down

implant
bent
up

If this implies that a man who wears a malleable prosthesis walks around with a kind of erection, so it should. He can, however, bend his penis up or down to whatever position he wants in order to use it. Also, the "hinged" prosthesis is easy to insert and avoids other medical complications.

It has been several years since I inserted a penile prosthesis in a prostate cancer patient. A patient's reaction to erectile dysfunction is never predictable, though, and I am forever surprised by it. For example, when one man wants to talk to me about a prosthesis with his partner in the background, the partner invariably signals, "Please! Please! Forget it!" Another wife, whose husband has recently battled prostate cancer and is impotent because of it, demands that her husband's sexual functions be fully restored. This is not always possible, but we urologists certainly try.

19. Prostate cancer: The aftereffects

One good thing about being a urologist at the outset of a new century is that, unlike the patients of other specialists, such as the cardiologist or neurosurgeon, relatively few of my patients will die from prostate problems, even though they may have been plagued by them for a long time.

It is also true that another U.S. survey showed how the happiest doctors practicing medicine today were urologists! I can only surmise that if this is correct, it is probably because most people are helped by urological interventions, whether they be treatments for an enlarged prostate or help with advanced prostate cancer.

Alas, some patients will have advanced prostate cancer for the balance of their lives, and the only consolation in this for me is that these men are usually quite elderly and will more likely die of other causes.

I have had failures, though. One was a fifty-year-old man who, like so many other patients, came to see me with a suspicious nodule on the left side of his prostate. The biopsy was positive for a Gleason Grade 7 cancer despite the fact the man's PSA reading was very low—only 1.4.

Within only three weeks of diagnosis he underwent a routine radical prostatectomy. The pathology on his prostate gland at that time confirmed a Gleason Grade 7 tumor, and one that was well confined. This, and the man's postoperative PSA readings— of almost zero—hinted that his problems may have been solved.

They were deceptive, though—especially when the patient complained of severe lower abdominal pains. Within a year after his surgery, a large lump where his prostate had been was readily palpable on rectal examination with my finger, and from then on his deterioration was swift. Despite aggressive radiotherapy, hormone therapy, and chemotherapy, this man died within two years of his radical prostatectomy—possibly because the early reoccurrence of his prostate cancer was not readily apparent.

Even in retrospect, I do not know what I—or my team—could have done differently. Sometimes, death is just due to the cruel hand of fate. Nonetheless, I have always felt that all men who have had prostate problems, no matter how mild or severe, should receive urological follow-ups on a regular basis.

Depending on a patient's medical history, follow-ups might include:
- regular, biannual PSA tests
- rectal examinations
- urinalysis
- routine history and physical examinations
- flow studies and cystoscopies for patients with continuing voiding problems
- ultrasound, bone scans, and CT scans for patients whose PSA readings are rising dramatically

As I've tried to stress, a PSA blood test remains the best marker not only for diagnosing prostate cancer, but for following the progress of a patient after a radical prostatectomy or radiotherapy. If his count remains near zero after these treatments, he can be considered cured.

If there are incremental rises in a patient's PSA on each of three six-month tests, a local recurrence of his tumor is suspected. A biopsy can then be tried again, but for a man who has had a prostatectomy it is usually not helpful. There is, after all, no prostate gland to target. For a recurrence following radiotherapy I prescribe hormone treatment; for a patient who still has cancer after a prostatectomy, I suggest a course of radiotherapy targeted to where his prostate once was.

If there is a doubling of the PSA count every six months, I suspect something more serious—a systemic spread of the cancer. In this case I put the patient on cyclical hormonal therapy, which could last indefinitely.

It would be wonderful if we had a scan that could tell us exactly where a tumor reoccurs, but we don't. The next best thing is the ProstaScint, a scan test that is meant to tell us where the PSA-secreting cells are by illuminating them rather like a bone scan does. There are, however, too many false positives and false negatives to make it consistently useful. Besides, this test is prohibitively expensive, with each one costing about $2,600.

More controversial than the ProstaScint scan test is what we call the RT-PCR PSA test. The abbreviation stands for "reverse transcriptase polymerase chain reaction." This test also attempts to identify PSA-secreting cells, but only those in the circulating blood. A positive test result before a radical prostatectomy should indicate that live prostate cancer cells are already in the blood circulation, making surgery futile. A positive result after surgery or radiotherapy, however, might indicate a failure of these treatments as well.

But again, there are too many false positives and false negatives to make the RT-RCR PSA test meaningful, and it has been abandoned in clinical practice.

The need for meticulous follow-up is well illustrated by yet another of my patients, a fifty-nine-year-old accountant. On his first visit to my office this man had only a mild obstruction of his urine flow. On rectal examination, the left side of his prostate felt firmer than the right. A biopsy of the firm area was done, but it was negative for cancer. One year later, however, a repeat biopsy revealed a Gleason Grade 7 cancer, and by this time the man's PSA reading was 10.7.

Soon afterward, I performed a radical prostatectomy on him, and the pathology report on the removed prostate revealed extensive cancer in the left lobe—a tumor that was approaching, but not invading, the edges of the tissue. In other words, this man's cancer was on the verge of escaping from the gland.

Subsequent biannual PSA blood test levels were close to zero for four years, but then they started to rise. Within a further four years they had gone from 0.7 to a worrisome 4.6, but the patient had no ill effects whatsoever. He urinated well and was able to have an erection.

Nonetheless, I decided that his cancer had reoccurred, and I treated him accordingly with hormones—Casodex to block testosterone from entering the prostate cells, and Zolodex to stop the testicles from making it. I was happy to see his PSA fall to 0.2.

When I stopped this treatment, however, the patient's PSA shot up again—to 1.4. At this point, he and I decided on a bone scan, which was negative. Radiotherapy to the prostate bed was then agreed upon, and after its completion the patient's PSA dropped back to below 1. Today, eleven years after his prostatectomy, his PSA is still low and—more important—he is enjoying his life.

This case illustrates several points. It is not unusual for patients who are seemingly cured and have zero PSAs to suddenly see their PSA levels rise some years after having had surgery. It is also not unusual for such a patient to respond to hormone therapy or radiotherapy. In fact, we might even ask: Would he have been better off without the surgery in the first place? Or is he better off today because of the surgery? The answer, of course, is that we don't really know.

What we are more sure about is that even if a patient is not cured by surgery—and it is naive to think that everyone will be—the progression of his disease will not necessarily be accelerated. Only on rare occasions do patients in whom cancer cells are left suffer a disturbing progression of their tumors like a fire out of control.

There are two schools of thought about which patients should have radical prostatectomies and which shouldn't. At the moment, these operations are generally confined to healthy men who, as we have discussed, are under seventy, have early confined disease, and have ten good years of life ahead of them.

Some urologists, like Dr. Thomas Stamey, believe that if the prostate is more than 40 percent invaded by a tumor, there is no point in removing it because a cure may be impossible. Dr. Alan Partin reinforces this view with an elaborate table that gives odds for the likelihood of a surgical cure based on different levels of PSA readings combined with different designations of the Gleason Grade.

These doctors feel that by making a man undergo surgery that may not be curative, his general well-being will be compromised as he struggles to recover. It would be better, they say, to supplant surgery with radio and/or hormone therapy almost immediately after the tumor has been found to be extensive.

Other doctors, however—particularly those at the Mayo Clinic, in Rochester, Minnesota—hold an opposite view. They think that denying a patient a prostatectomy because his cancer may be locally extensive, and relying solely on hormone treatment and radiotherapy, is somehow accepting that surgery has no role to play in prolonging life when a tumor may be advanced.

I agree with that. I feel strongly that it is wrong to administer only palliative-type treatment so soon after diagnosis, and that the radical prostatectomy has a role for *many* cancer patients regardless of how extensive their tumors may be. Surgery may not actually rid a man of all of his cancer, of course. This is something we won't know, even following pathology reports during and after the operation itself—the cancer may well have spread.

That problem is conceded. Radical surgery will, however, help the patient alleviate any urinary problems he may suffer later because his cancerous prostate may be enlarged. It may even prevent kidney damage and the severe, unrelenting pain that this incurs.

There is also a strong psychological yearning in all patients to be completely rid of an organ that is harboring cancer, especially one—like the prostate—that has such a limited use anyway and is so capable of holding a tumor for such a long time.

Finally on this point, we must remind ourselves once more that while hormone treatment can be given at any time, surgery cannot follow any radiotherapy that may have failed. Radiotherapy, however, can—and must—be given when cancer recurs after surgery.

Admittedly, there have been many cases when, in hindsight, a radical prostatectomy may have been unnecessary. Against this, there is no defense. When there are overwhelming indications of cancer we have no alternative but to surge ahead. I once treated a man who was seventy in whom an early prostate tumor was diagnosed. I proposed a curative radical prostatectomy, but the patient had other ideas. He wanted to delay the procedure until he had completed psychiatric treatment for depression. In the interim he agreed to hormonal treatment—until his psychiatrist persuaded him to go for the surgery.

To my surprise, when the prostate was removed the pathologist couldn't find any cancer. I was stunned and, fearing a misdiagnosis, promptly rechecked the biopsy I had taken before the operation. Lo and behold, cancer had been there all right, but it was now gone! I suspect that the patient's tumor was among that rare 4 percent completely eradicated by hormone treatment.

When patients are no longer helped by hormones, further treatment depends upon their overall health. If a man is bedridden and in severe pain, no attempts are made to fight the cancer. From then on, his treatment truly is palliative. Pain control and cortisone preparations, along with a drug called Mitoxantrone (between 12 and 14 mg per square meter of body surface every three weeks), are all that will be prescribed for him. Mitoxantrone has been demonstrated to help alleviate pain, and although no cures can be attributed to it, it may lengthen lives.

Palliative radiotherapy

If the pain from prostate cancer in the bones is well localized, spot-radiation to the site is very effective for symptomatic relief. There may be increased pain for two to three days immediately after the radiation—ironically a sign of good results—and then complete relief after one or two weeks. Happily, I can report that palliative radiation controls pain in between 80 and 90 percent of patients.

Radiation that is not for cure, but for the relief of symptoms, has also been used when a tumor has collapsed a vertebrae and the spinal cord or nerve roots are compressed. It is effective, too, when there is urinary bleeding, a blockage in a ureter, or a distressing pain deep in the lower abdomen, at the site of the prostate.

When there is extensive cancer in the backbone, or vertebral body, it can collapse and shorten the bone, and, at the same time, expand one of the cartilaginous discs that lie between the vertebrae. This expansion places pressure on the spinal cord, causing severe pain that brings on neurological signs or symptoms.

Patients say they feel "electric shocks" in their legs, increased sensations to slight touches, lessened sensations or numbness, or even paralysis. The collapse of the bone and the protrusion of the disc can be diagnosed by a nuclear magnetic scan, or by a CT scan combined with a dye that is injected into the spinal canal in a procedure known as a myelogram.

If such a patient is not already on hormonal therapy, this is started immediately. Because of its fast action, Ketoconazole, an antifungal agent, may be the treatment of choice. Then, radiotherapy is begun.

Neurosurgical intervention (nerve decompression) is considered if the spine is unstable, when there is neurological deterioration while the patient is on radiotherapy, or when he suffers nerve compression to areas that were previously radiated. Often, this kind of surgery—a judgment call—is performed by neurosurgeons or orthopedic surgeons.

Radiotherapy for nerve compression not only relieves the pain in more than 90 percent of cases, but improves the neurological status in about two-thirds of them. The treatment to control bleeding, to open up a blocked ureter, or to provide relief for patients with intractable pelvic distress is often tried, usually out of desperation, but there are only occasional happy outcomes.

Palliative pain control

Pain management has become a specialized art. Doctors involved in palliative—often terminal—care provide most of the expertise. They utilize various combinations of drugs, starting with codeine, progressing to Duragesic (fentanyl) or Percocet (oxycodone), and finally graduating to the better-known morphine and dilaudid.

Many of these drugs are formulated to be long-acting so that they only need to be taken twice a day. Shorter-acting drugs are used to establish the right dosage. Ten milligrams of morphine by injection, or 20 to 30 milligrams by mouth, will control pain for between three and four hours. The equivalent dose for codeine is 120 milligrams by injection or 180 to 240 milligrams by mouth; for Percocet, the equivalent dosage is 15 milligrams by injection, 10 to 15 milligrams by mouth; and for dilaudid, 2 milligrams by injection or between 20 and 30 milligrams by mouth.

Duragesic, which is sold as a skin patch containing fentanyl, comes in four different strengths and the effects of each patch last three days.

In addition to pain-controlling medications, bowel softeners such as Colace (docusate), laxatives like Senokot (senna), and antinausea preparations like Maxeran (metoclopramide) can be very helpful to make patients more comfortable. Mental agitation, hallucinations, and delusional thoughts that precede death are best treated with 5 milligrams of Haldol (haloperidol) three times a day.

Toxic chemotherapy

If patients with advanced prostate cancer are walking, vigorous, and otherwise well, different chemotherapy protocols may be considered. Toxic chemotherapy regimes have been pioneered by Dr. Ken Pienta in Detroit, by Dr. Howard Scher at Memorial Sloan-Kettering, by Dr. Dan Petrylak at New York's Columbia Presbyterian Medical Center, and by oncologists at the M.D. Anderson Institute in Houston, Texas, among many others.

Pienta's regime consists of the drug Emcyt (estramustine phosphate) given—in a dosage of one 140-milligram tablet for every twenty-five to thirty pounds (11 to 14 kg) of body weight—three or four times a day. This drug is combined with Velbe (vinblastine sulfate) and administered intravenously once a week for six weeks at the rate of 4 milligrams for every square meter of body surface. In another regime, Vepesid (etoposide) taken orally (50 mg twice daily) substitutes for the intravenous Velbe.

During toxic chemotherapy, patients must be closely monitored and their treatments interrupted when or if their white cell counts drop below 2,000. Half of these patients respond with lower PSA readings, and an actual control of prostate cancer has been observed in a few instances.

The M.D. Anderson group has used Ketoconazole with Adriamycin (doxorubicin) with similar results. The Ketoconazole dosage is usually 1,200 milligrams orally per day, while the daily dosage of Adriamycin is between 60 and 75 milligrams per square meter of body surface.

Usually, patients who require chemotherapy are sent to the oncologist. Some time ago, however, I decided to administer toxic chemotherapy to ten patients I had been tending for many years myself. All had developed "hormone-independent" cancer and were frightened of the consequences. All were also reluctant to see other doctors, feeling that if I suggested they did so, they were being abandoned.

All ten men were in good shape, up and about, and limited only by the distress the advancing disease had caused them. I put them all on Emcyt (roughly 10 milligrams per kilogram of body weight) and Vepesid (50 milligrams twice a day), and monitored their white blood counts weekly. The health of three of the ten men improved and there was a corresponding fall in their PSA levels, but the demise of two men was accelerated.

I am not certain whether I helped or worsened the conditions of the remaining five patients. I was not impressed with the effects of toxic chemotherapy, nor with my role in their care. I now refer all my hormone-failing patients to an oncologist without allowing them to persuade me otherwise.

Experimental therapy

For now, some therapies for prostate problems are far too experimental to be used—even as backups when all other treatments have failed. If they turn out to be worthwhile, however, they may well replace hormone therapy, radiotherapy, and even surgery as the definite treatments.

These new therapies are:

- angiogenesis inhibitors
- gene therapy
- immunotherapy

Angiogenesis inhibitors are pills predicated on the assumption that cancer cells need fresh blood to nourish them. Thus, it follows that if we prevent new blood vessels from forming near a cluster of cancer cells, the tumor will be starved and killed.

This effort, which has progressed from the laboratory to test trials, has been pioneered by Dr. Judah Folkman in Boston. Several products are in phase-three trials and are expected on the market within the next two years.

Gene therapy is also still experimental but equally as promising as the angiogenesis inhibitors. Put simply, the cancerous prostate is injected with a virus that can be killed by a specific drug. The virus thrives and multiplies within the cancer cells, and, after sufficient time, when it has incorporated itself as part of the cancer, it is killed off. In the process, the cancer cells die, too.

In another version, a genetically modified virus is injected into the prostate. This thrives specifically in cancer cells that produce PSA. Eventually, the altered DNA kills those cells by preventing them from multiplying.

In experimental immunotherapy, cancer cells extracted from the patient's prostate are irradiated—by X-rays—so they cannot multiply but remain able to retain their collective ability to trigger an immune response. These cells are incubated with protein-processing cells (called dendritic cells), which are grown outside the body. The cells are then injected back into the patient's bloodstream where, ideally, they trigger an immune response.

In summary, angiogenesis inhibitors, gene therapy, and immunotherapy are promising leads in the fight against prostate cancer.

What about PC-Spes?

When I was in Beijing, China, in 1982, where I was participating in a medical symposium, I saw a baby delivered by cesarean section when the only anesthetic used was acupuncture! I was dumbfounded.

Later that day, I asked the gynecologist in charge of the procedure whether acupuncture could be used to change bad habits, like smoking, drinking, and gambling. She laughed aloud and said, "Acupuncture is a form of analgesia—perhaps 70 percent as effective as a general anesthetic. Why would you think it can change a bad habit?"

This was an embarrassing exchange for me. Perhaps I should have known more about acupuncture. But it set me thinking. I immediately thought that if acupuncture could alleviate the pain of a cesarean section, there's no reason why it couldn't have an application in certain corners of urology. This, I have not yet explored; what I do know, though, is that there are treatments in Asia that are as yet untried in the West, and, given time, they may well find a place in conventional medicine.

One of these may well be PC-Spes—a herbal concoction prepared from chrysanthemum petals, isatis, licorice, lucid ganaderma, pseudo-ginseng, rubescens, saw palmetto, and scute. In limited trials throughout the United States, PC-Spes appears to lower the PSA counts of patients with advanced prostate cancer—men who are no longer responding to hormone therapy. It is reasonably nontoxic, and patients taking the preparation feel fine.

The mystery is this: How does it work?

The theory is that PC-Spes may simply interfere with the action of the bel-2 gene, thus promoting apoptosis, or programmed cell death. It may work best when combined with other cancer-killing drugs. At best, it is an intriguing product and we shall have to wait to see if it is for real. We must await the results of a wider trial.

On a more conventional front, diverse efforts to overcome prostate cancer have attracted the attention of scientists from around the world, and Canadian contributions have been significant. Dr. Charles Huggins, a Canadian, was working in Chicago when he made his Nobel Prize–winning studies on the effects of male hormones on prostate cancer—that testosterone was guilty of promoting it, and eliminating testosterone could be helpful. Dr. Fernand Labrie, of Quebec City, later studied a family of drugs called antiandrogens, and how they halt the production of testosterone from the adrenal gland and block it from entering prostate cancer cells.

I have mentioned Dr. Joe Chin as one of the pioneers in cryosurgery, and Dr. John Trachtenberg as an ardent believer in thermal ablation. I should, however, also tell you that in Vancouver, Dr. Nicholas Bruchovsky and Dr. Larry Goldenberg have done important work. These men pioneered the idea that intermittent hormone therapy may be more effective than continuous hormone therapy—and be better tolerated by the patient in the bargain.

The next Canadian breakthrough in the treatment of prostate cancer may well come from Dr. Martin Gleave, one of Dr. Goldenberg's associates at the University of British Columbia, or from my colleagues, Dr. Mostafa Elhilali, Dr. Armen Aprikian, Dr. Simone Chevalier, Dr. Mario Chevrette, and Dr. Simon Tanguay, at McGill University. I cannot, however, ignore the diagnostics research being done by Dr. Yves Fradet and his team at l'Université Laval in Quebec City and by Dr. Fred Saad and his associates at the University of Montreal, nor Dr. Larry Klotz's valuable work at the University of Toronto. The Vancouver group may be advantaged on this front, though, because it has recently received a generous grant from a local entrepreneur.

The bottom line: a consumer advocate

Reduce your risks for developing prostate cancer. Take antioxidants, like vitamins C and E, selenium, lycopenes, and glutathione. Soy products won't hurt, either. Cut down on animal fats, especially those found in red meat and butter. Exercise, and stay mentally upbeat.

Find a kind but competent doctor who will not object to ordering annual PSA tests following each rectal examination.

Know your PSA level in numbers and do not accept "It was okay" as a complete answer. Get a transrectal ultrasound and sextant biopsy (those six needles) whenever the PSA is too high or the rectal examination is abnormal. Ask for a copy of the biopsy report.

If cancer is found, see how it is rated according to Dr. Partin's table, then do the following:

- Think long and hard before deciding on a radical prostatectomy, conformal radiotherapy, or brachytherapy.
- Ask for hormone treatment before radiotherapy but preferably not before surgery.
- Do not neglect your follow-ups.
- Insist on a PSA reading at least every six months.
- Keep your eyes and ears open for new developments, such as PC-Spes, angiogenesis inhibitors, gene therapy, and immunotherapy.
- Be leery of toxic chemotherapy but welcome Mitoxantrone and cortisone if necessary.
- Never second-guess any decision you make.

Above all, try to look on the bright side and remember that a cheerful, optimistic patient is more likely to be properly managed in his battle with prostate cancer than a sad and angry one.

Glossary

Acini: The secreting portion of glands.

Antimicrobial: A product that kills or stops the reproduction of bacteria.

Autosomal chromosome: A chromosome that is not an X or Y sex chromosome.

Balloon dilation: Stretching open the urethra running through the prostate by inflating a balloon attached to a modified Foley catheter that is placed in the urethra.

Benign prostatic hyperplasia: A non-malignant growth of prostate tissue occurring after middle age, often associated with disturbances in urine flow.

Bone scan: X-ray like imaging of the skeleton after injection of a radioactive tracer that can reveal the presence of cancer in bones.

Brachytherapy: Radiotherapy by implantation of radioactive seeds into cancerous organs like the prostate.

Cell differentiation: The extent of architectural changes in cancer cells when compared to the normal.

c-erb B2: A tumor promoting gene that works on growth promoting signals.

Combination therapy: The use of more than one modality of treatment, such as surgery and radiotherapy.

Computerized tomogram scan (CT scan): X-rays directed at the body that are made to form a picture as if the body were guillotined at different levels, 0.5 to 1 cm apart.

Cunningham clamp: A padded clamp with different settings that squeezes the urethra from front to back, stopping the continuous leakage of urine.

Cystoscopy: A direct inspection of the lining of the urethra and bladder lining by means of an instrument fitted with a lens at one end and fiberoptic lighting at the other end.

Dendritic cells: Cells located in skin, as well as elsewhere, that process foreign proteins, like cancer cells, rendering them capable of inducing an immune response.

Dihydrotestosterone: A male hormone five times more powerful than testosterone.

E-cadherin: A molecule that normally binds cells together and that is regulated by a specific gene.

Experimental immunotherapy: Immunotherapy techniques that have yet to become established in clinical practice.

Flow study: A measurement, depicted on a graph, of the amount of urine passed per unit of time. The maximum flow rate and the total amount of urine voided are also noted.

Free radical: A molecule containing an unpaired electron in its outer orbit. Free radicals may cause effects such as DNA damage, which may promote cancer.

Holmium laser: An example of a short–wave length laser that can carve out relatively large glands without any significant blood loss.

Hyperthermia treatment: Heating the prostate as if by placing it in a microwave oven.

Impotence: The inability to have an erection sufficient for sexual intercourse, now called erectile dysfunction.

Incontinence: The involuntary loss of urine.

Intravenous pyelogram: A diagnostic test in which a liquid contrast material, which in an X-ray shows up like bone, is injected intravenously and is depicted by sequential X-rays as it is excreted from the kidneys and drainage system.

Kegel exercise: Squeezing of the muscles used to stop the urine in mid-flow.

Laser energy: The term laser is an acronym derived from light amplification by stimulated emission of radiation. In effect, a laser beam, unlike a light beam, is much more focused and can create intense heat and destroy tissue with precision. The depth of tissue destruction is dependent upon the source material. Deep destruction occurs with short–wave length lasers, like argon and ruby, while shallow destruction occurs with long–wave length lasers, like YAG (yttrium-aluminum-garnet) or carbon dioxide.

Lycopene: The chemical that makes tomatoes and other foods, like watermelon, red and that may play a role in fighting prostate cancer.

Lymphocele: A collection of fluid within a lymphatic lining.

Metastases: Cancer spread located in distant sites.

Metastatic cancer: Cancer that has spread to distant sites.

Morsellator: A tool like a miniaturized meat grinder fashioned with a suction device to pull tissue into the contraption.

Neo-adjuvant therapy: Treatment such as hormonal therapy preceding definitive treatment like radiotherapy or surgery.

Nuclear magnetic scan: Imaging like the CT scan but based on the principle that magnetic fields are deflected by the varying composition of human tissue.

Oncogenes: Genes that promote cancer.

P53: A tumor suppressor gene.

Palliative treatment: Treatment not meant to cure but to provide comfort and control of the disease.

Partin table: A table that predicts curability with radical prostatectomy based on the Gleason Grade and PSA.

Penis: The male organ of copulation and urinary excretion.

Ploidy analysis: Examination of the number of chromosomes within the cell nucleus; diploid usually signifies a less aggressive cancer with 46 chromosomes, while aneuploid signifies a more aggressive cancer with more than the usual 46 chromosomes.

Pressure-flow study: Examination of urine flow as it relates to the pressure generated by the bladder.

Priapism: Painful, undesired, and sustained erection resulting in a permanent loss of erection unless treated promptly.

Prostate: A male sex gland that produces the bulk of the fluid that comprises the semen.

Prostatic infarct: A blockage of one of the small arteries to the prostate, causing destruction of that part of the prostate vascularized by that vessel and associated with short-term high PSA readings.

Prostatic intraepithelial neoplasia (PIN): Non-cancerous but cancer-like changes in the nucleus of prostate gland cells that are read as low grade, which has no prognostic significance, and high grade, which is often pre-malignant.

Prostatic massage: Kneading, by a gloved, lubricated finger, of the prostate from side to middle and top to bottom to squeeze prostatic fluid from the gland into the urethra.

Ras proto-oncogene: A tumor promoting gene.

Resectoscope: An instrument, like a cystoscope, passed through the urethra to carve out prostate tissue.

Residual urine: The urine left behind in the bladder after urination.

Retinoblastoma gene: A tumor suppressor gene located on chromosome 13.

Retrograde or "dry" ejaculation: An ejaculation that produces no external discharge. The fluid shoots instead backwards into the bladder.

Retropubic prostatectomy: Finger enucleation of enlarged prostate tissue via an incision in the lower abdomen providing access to an area behind the pubic bone.

Scrotum: The pouch of skin that contains the testicles.

Seminal vesicles: A reproductive organ attached to the back of the prostate that makes part of the fluid that constitutes semen.

Stent: A hollow tube that is inserted into a passage to keep it open.

Stroma: the support structure of glands.

Testicles: The paired male reproductive glands within the scrotum that make testosterone and spermatozoa.

Testosterone: The quintessential male hormone.

Transitional zone of the prostate: The inner part of the prostate near the urethra where benign enlargement occurs. It is also the source of 15 to 20 percent of prostate cancers.

TURP syndrome: A life threatening condition caused by a massive absorption of irrigating fluid used in the process of carving out the prostate.

Ultrasound residual: The amount of urine left in the bladder after urination. measured by a device applied to the skin in the lower abdomen.

Uremia: Kidney failure characterized by accumulation of waste products in the blood and disturbances in chemical and acid balance.

Urodynamic study: A study of bladder function that is done by artificially filling and emptying the bladder and measuring pressures at different levels.

Urology: A surgical discipline that deals with urinary tract disorders in women and urinary tract and genital system disorders in men.

Watchful waiting: Monitoring cancer with periodic blood tests and clinical assessments rather than actively treating the disease.

Support Groups

There is an abundance of emotional and educational support available to men who are suffering from all manner of prostate problems, particularly cancer. Local support groups and organizations can usually be contacted through a general hospital, a urologist's office, or the following national support centers.

United States

Us Too International Inc.
930 North York Rd., Suite 50
Hinsdale, IL
60521-2993
(800) 80-USTOO
http://www.ustoo.com/

Patient Advocates for
Advanced Cancer Treatment
(PAACT)
1143 Parmelee, NW
Grand Rapids, MI
49504
(616) 453-1477
http://www.prostatepointers.
org/paact/

Man to Man
c/o American Cancer Society
1599 Clinton Rd., NE
Atlanta, GA
30329
(800) ACS-2345
http://www.cancer.org/
m2m.htm/

The Educational Center for
Prostate Cancer Patients
(ECPCP)
P.O. Box 948
Westbury, NY
11590
(516) 997-1777
http://www.ecpcp.org/

Canada

Canadian Cancer Society
Cancer Information Service
(888) 939-3333
http://www.cancer.ca

Index

antiandrogens, 136–137
bilateral orchiectomy, 134
combination treatment, 137–138,
    202
components, 132
cyclical hormonal therapy, 138
erectile dysfunction, 166
female hormone pill, 134–135
"flare," 136
incontinence, 166
medical castration, 135–136
Nizoral, 134
objective, 132
subcapsular orchiectomy, 134
vs. surgical castration, 138–139
and unrelated health problems,
    133
*How I Survived Prostate Cancer ...
    And So Can You* (Lewis), 7
Huggins, Charles, 198
hyperthermia treatment, 79–80, 144,
    202
Hytrin, 37, 65, 84

I

imaging techniques, 17
imipramine, 169
immune system, 97–98
immunotherapy, 197
impotence. *See* erectile dysfunction
impregnation, 13
Imuran, 78
incontinence, 149, 167–172, 202
    bladder-muscle thickening,
        167–168
    cystoscopy, 169
    hormone treatment, 166
    Kegel exercises, 168
    radiotherapy, 166
    sphincter damage, 169–171
Indocid, 82, 83
indomethacin, 82
International Prostate Symptom
    Score (IPSS), 30–31, 64–65
Internet information, 87–88, 148
interstitial cystitis, 84–85
intravenous antibiotics, 72

intravenous pyelogram, 21, 203
isoflavones, 101

J

Japan, 101–102
Johnson, Virginia, 172

K

Kefzol, 72
Kegel exercises, 150, 168, 203
Ketoconazole, 134, 195
Kettering, Sloan, 195
kidneys, 58–59, 64
"kissing" lobes, 21
klebsiella, 71
Klotz, Larry, 199
Korda, Michael, 7

L

Labrie, Fernand, 198–199
laser energy, 53–54, 145, 203
Lepor, Herbert, 150
Levoquin, 78
Lewis, James, 7
Leydid cells, 27
lifestyles, 27, 65, 98, 101–103
Living with Prostate Cancer
    (Newton), 7
lower urinary tract symptoms
    (LUTS), 29
Lupron, 136
LUTS. *See* lower urinary tract
    symptoms (LUTS)
lycopene, 102, 203
lymph nodes, 99
lymphocele, 203

M

Ma prostate chérie (Delbuguet), 7
Man to Man: Surviving Prostate
    Cancer (Korda), 7
Masters, William, 172
Maxeran, 194
Mayo Clinic, 190
M.D. Anderson Institute, 195
Meares, Edwin, 76
medical castration, 135–136